AF477993

BETSY L. BARR

Associate Editor
Lahey Clinic Foundation
Boston, Massachusetts

SURGERY OF THE VULVA AND VAGINA
A Practical Guide

EDWARD H. COPENHAVER, M.D.

Chairman, Department of Gynecology
Lahey Clinic Foundation
Boston, Massachusetts

PAUL D. MALONE

FRANCIS E. STECKEL

ANNE S. GREENE

Department of Medical Illustration
Lahey Clinic Foundation
Boston, Massachusetts

1981   W. B. SAUNDERS COMPANY   Philadelphia London Toronto Sydney

W. B. Saunders Company: West Washington Square
Philadelphia, PA   19105

1 St. Anne's Road
Eastbourne, East Sussex BN21 3UN, England

1 Goldthorne Avenue
Toronto, Ontario M8Z 5T9, Canada

9 Waltham Street
Artarmon, N.S.W. 2064, Australia

Library of Congress Cataloging in Publication Data

Copenhaver, Edward H.

Surgery of vulva and vagina.

1. Vulva—Surgery.   2. Vagina—Surgery.   I. Title.
   [DNLM: 1. Vulva—Surgery.   2. Vagina—Surgery.
   WP200 C782s]

RG104.C58   618.1'5059   80-51958

ISBN 0-7216-2718-8

Surgery of the Vulva and Vagina   ISBN   0-7216-2718-8

Last digit is the print number: 9   8   7   6   5   4   3   2   1

Preface

The purpose of this book is to present in concise form the surgical methods employed and preferred by the surgical author. Such methodology is not static but changes in response to experience here and elsewhere. Few current surgical techniques have survived unchanged over the past two decades.

Mr. Paul D. Malone, Mr. Francis E. Steckel, and Mrs. Anne S. Greene of the Department of Medical Illustration of the Lahey Clinic Foundation are coauthors, thereby emphasizing the working partnership that must exist between surgeon and artist in such an endeavor.

Most of the minor procedures described should be part of the armamentarium of all physicians who treat women, for they form the basis for early detection of disease and management of minor problems. Culdoscopy, however, is rarely used at the present time except when laparoscopy equipment fails or when a free cul-de-sac exists in the presence of severe midabdominal adhesions. Hysteroscopy is considered a research technique at the present time and therefore is not included. The use of the laser beam also is not discussed because of its current status as a research technique.

In regard to the recommended suture material, it is important that each physician employ the sutures with which he or she is familiar. In general, while the synthetic absorbable suture is stronger and creates less tissue reaction than catgut, a special technique is required to tie the knots. We have been inclined to use chromic catgut whenever there is much tension on the suture line.

We have avoided unnecessary references but have made note in the text of the originator of a technique when it has not been significantly altered. However, selected references are given when appropriate, especially in the section on radical surgery of the vulva because of the controversy surrounding its clinical management.

EDWARD H. COPENHAVER, M.D.

Special appreciation is extended to my secretaries, Mrs. Patricia Osgood Tipping and Mrs. Dorothy Crispo, and to my wife, Margaret, and my daughter, Jane, for many hours of extra work on this project; and special thanks go to our nurses, Mrs. Philomena Murray, Mrs. Kathleen Walker, and Mrs. Elaine Hartwell, for their help regarding technical details.

We are grateful to Ms. Betsy L. Barr of the Editorial Department and to the W. B. Saunders Company for their roles in transforming our work into a readable text.

Contents

General Considerations

INTRODUCTION

PHILOSOPHIC AND PSYCHOLOGIC CONSIDERATIONS

Philosophic

The surgeon should pause periodically for a sober reexamination of his or her surgical policies. When the benefits and risks of current therapy are counterbalanced, the benefits should decisively outweigh the risks. If they do not, then the surgeon's philosophy of practice should be modified to fit the facts. Physicians are constantly weighing the good and bad points of a treatment policy to arrive at the best course of action for the individual patient. We must avoid taking an overzealous approach to surgical treatment without first weighing the risks involved.

What is a surgeon's philosophy of gynecologic surgery? Will the surgeon subject the patient to a more extensive operative procedure than is necessary, at increased morbidity and mortality rates? When the patient requires contraceptive advice, will the physician suggest vaginal hysterectomy and repair or sterilization for the patient or her husband? Will mild stress incontinence of urine be magnified into an indication for vaginal hysterectomy and repair? Will the surgeon take a simplistic approach to treatment of preinvasive and invasive malignancy of the vulva or tailor the extent of operation to the clinical and pathologic findings of the individual patient?

Such philosophic considerations bring into focus the question of necessary versus unnecessary surgery. If necessary surgery were defined as that which removes the patient from a life-threatening medical problem, much of major gynecologic surgery must be considered unnecessary. On the other hand, if necessary surgery were defined as any procedure that enhances the physical and mental well-being of a patient, gynecologic surgery would have a broader base of indications. With this second definition, the vast majority of hysterectomies would fall into the category of "necessary."

By contrast, most of the procedures for vaginal relaxation, prolapse, and stress incontinence should be labeled "unnecessary."

When a life-threatening situation is not involved, the risks and the benefits of surgery should be discussed with the patient, so that she may be a partner in the decision for or against operation. To this end, the author would favor liberal consultation. Because both physicians and patients honestly lack respect for the risks of operation, I do not believe that the numbers of operations will be reduced except through compulsory consultation. Consultants should not perform the operation but remain neutral judges.

Admittedly, reduction of "unnecessary surgery" is not a simple task. It places an increased burden on the judgment and diagnostic skills of the physician. Despite the prudent use of colposcopy, biopsy, examination under anesthesia, curettage, and laparoscopy, diagnostic errors will increase slightly. Therefore, we occasionally must resort to laparotomy and even hysterectomy in the face of intractable, unexplained pelvic symptoms.

Psychologic

When the past 25 years of my association with many gynecologic surgeons in six hospitals is reviewed, it becomes evident that too little attention has been given to the environmental and inner tensions that influence the outcome of a surgical procedure. Pressures created by an unrealistic schedule, by nervous or unhappy associates, and by preoccupations of the surgeon with other problems may result in poor or hasty judgment at the operating table. A serene operating room and competent surgical nurse have much to do with the quality of surgery.

Speed at the operating table too often has been equated with surgical skill. When such speed reflects a masterful organization of surgical techniques, it may be an asset. However, too often such speed reflects the need to meet a later appointment, a desire to impress younger physicians and nurses, or just the inner restlessness of the surgeon. It is believed that uncontrolled speed at the operating table is the foremost cause of surgical complications.

Fatigue of the surgeon and major surgery are a bad combination. If a surgeon has been obliged to go without rest for a long time, it may be wise to defer an operation. If an extensive, radical, or tedious operation is to be performed, it is better to start such a procedure early in the morning when the operating team is physically and mentally alert.

A depressed or anxious or emotionally unstable person breeds disaster in the operating room. Psychologic well-being of the operating room team and good surgery go hand in hand.

PREOPERATIVE EVALUATION AND CARE

Preoperative and postoperative evaluation and care at the Lahey Clinic involve liberal use of medical consultants, for it is better to prevent a medical or surgical complication than to manage one. The basic history of a patient should include in the following order: age, parity, chief complaint and its duration, present illness, any family history of diabetes mellitus, cancer, or cardiovascular disease, and the patient's history of allergy, cough, chest pain, shortness of breath, intestinal upset, urinary symptoms, serious illness, and operations. The physical examination should include recording of the temperature and blood pressure, notation of any loose teeth or dentures, palpation of the thyroid gland and lymph nodes, auscultation of the heart and lungs, palpation of the breasts and abdomen, a bimanual pelvic and rectal examination, and notation of any lower extremity edema or varicosities.

Supplementary studies before anesthesia should include a complete blood cell count, blood glucose test, and urinalysis, a chest radiograph, and, for patients over age 40, an electrocardiogram. If major surgery is contemplated, a chemical and electrolyte profile of the blood may be added. Intravenous pyelography must be obtained if the nature of a pelvic mass is uncertain and if the patient has a history of recurrent urinary incontinence or infection.

Urologic consultation is obtained for patients with recurrent urinary tract infections and recurrent urinary incontinence. Consultation with the colon and rectal service and a barium enema examination are requested when a patient has a history of rectal bleeding. A surgical consultation and mammogram are obtained in the presence of a questionable finding on breast examination. Beyond this, medical opinion is sought for any significant abnormality encountered during the history taking and physical examination. The medical specialist not only evaluates the patient before anesthesia and operation but also observes postoperatively the patient with asthma, diabetes mellitus, serious hypertension, cardiovascular insufficiency, respiratory disease, or a history of phlebitis and embolism. Vaginitis should be treated before operation.

Although the genital area is shaved before major vaginal surgery, it is unnecessary to shave it before minor procedures unless such procedures directly involve the vulva. At the time of operation, the vagina and vulva are thoroughly scrubbed twice with povidone-iodine (Betadine) and rinsed with water. Povidone-iodine solution is applied again to the vagina and appropriate skin areas for a wide margin around the operative site. In patients undergoing major vaginal surgery, the anal area is covered with a plastic drape (3M small towel Steri-Drape No. 1000–12 × 18 inches or 30.5 × 46 cm) before the routine drapes are applied. Sterile towels are placed on each side of the genital area, forming a triangular operative site. If a concomitant suprapubic procedure is contemplated, this area is also prepared, and a third towel is used to cover the midabdomen.

An antibiotic program is begun just before operation and is continued for 72 hours after operation if an extensive operative dissection has been performed, if excessive blood has been lost, if dead space remains that may be a source of abscess formation, if an infection would jeopardize the result of the operation, if major vaginal surgery is performed, or if the medical status of the patient warrants administration of antibiotics. Antibiotic treatment consists of sodium cephalothin (Keflin), 1 gm given intravenously during operation and 1 gm (in 100 cc saline) given intravenously every six hours for 24 hours or as long as the intravenous fluids are continued, followed by cephalexin monohydrate (Keflex), 500 mg by mouth every six hours for 48 hours. Should the patient have an allergy to this drug or to penicillin, intramuscular tetracycline, 100 mg, is started before operation and continued every eight hours, after which oral tetracycline, 500 mg every six hours, may be given for a total of 72 hours after operation.

COMPLICATIONS AND MANAGEMENT

PREVENTION

Complications cannot be avoided, but they certainly may be reduced. It is far better to prevent a complication than it is to treat one. At the risk of redundancy, the following points will be reiterated:

1. Avoid unnecessary surgery. Do not be pushed into elective or irrational surgery by an unstable patient. Nothing is worse than to have a major complication or a death after an operation that was not indicated in the first place.

2. Evaluate medical problems and seek consultation *before* operation. This is important in patients with a history of cardiorespiratory symptoms. Patients should be cautioned against smoking before and after operation; Mattingly (1977) reported that pulmonary complications were a major cause in 30 per cent of postoperative deaths.

3. Maintain adequate hydration. Intravenous fluids should be given before operation to prevent dehydration in the patient with a history of bronchitis or asthma; however, beware of overhydrating the elderly patient and the patient with a history of heart failure. Gray (1966) encouraged the use of Ringer's lactate solution during and for 24 hours after operation.

4. Try to reduce the tendency toward serious thromboembolism. Mattingly (1977) reflected the current concept that phlebothrombosis and embolism are common after operation, with a continuous process of embolization and lysis occurring within the pulmonary circulation. Consider employing heparin (5,000 units subcutaneously twice daily beginning 12 hours before operation) in the presence of obesity, malignancy, varicose veins, previous history of embolism, severe diabetes, arteriosclerotic heart disease, cardiac failure, chronic pulmonary disease, and radical vulvectomy (at highest risk). Have the patient's legs elevated, encourage moving of the legs, and have the patient avoid sitting upright in bed or a chair.

5. Be constantly aware of the rectum, the bladder, and the ureters. Symmonds (1979) campaigned vigorously during the past decade to prevent genitourinary fistulas by encouraging awareness, adequate exposure, recognition of injury at operation, and avoidance of blind clamping in the presence of bleeding.

Beyond emphasis on prevention, the purpose of this section is to discuss surgical complications and management.

HEMORRHAGE

Much individual variation exists in amounts of operative and postoperative bleeding. In general, young patients with a better blood supply bleed more than postmenopausal patients. While vasoconstricting agents may reduce initial bleeding, thus improving exposure, they do not prevent serious bleeding problems. All surgeons should naturally be alert to the rare patient with a bleeding disorder. Excessive bleeding and transfusions are the rule with radical surgery for malignancy of the vulva. Reports on vaginal hysterectomy with and without repair provide some insight into the bleeding problem with vaginal surgery.

Transfusion rates vary from a low of 2.7 per cent (Amirikia and Evans, 1979) to 13 per cent (Ledger and Child, 1973). *Immediate hemorrhage* led to laparotomy in eight of 1,218 cases reported by Pratt and Scherman in 1954 (three from ovarian vessels, two from uterine vessels, and one each from the broad ligament, cervicopubic fascia, and vaginal mucosa); in four of 1,000 patients reported by me in 1962 (three from ovarian vessels, one from adnexal vessels with pelvic adhesions); and in three of 810 cases reported by Gray in 1966. *Excessive postoperative bleeding* occurred in 28 of 1,218 cases reported by Pratt and Scherman (nine required packs and two required sutures), 29 of 1,000 patients in my report (11 required packs and eight required clamps or sutures), and 12 of 810 cases reported by Gray (four required packs and eight required sutures).

The need for laparotomy can be avoided by performing a repair alone or a Manchester operation instead of vaginal hysterectomy. When hemorrhage occurs, pressure should be applied and then careful clamping and ligature attempted rather than wide and blind clamping. It is better to lose a pint of blood than to risk injury to the ureters, bladder, or rectum. It is also better to pack the vagina and perform a laparotomy than to risk serious injury.

In the case of postoperative vaginal bleeding, the surgeon should observe first, pack second, and return the patient to the operating room for clamping, suturing, or laparotomy as a last resort. In the presence of any excessive postoperative bleeding it is wise to maintain a catheter in the bladder, even when prudent observation is in order. The genital area should be cleansed thoroughly and prepared with a disinfectant solution before a large sterile gauze pack is inserted. It is better to clamp a bleeding vessel and leave the clamp or clamps in the vagina for two days than to tear friable tissue

and extend the hemorrhage with difficult suturing of the bleeding site.

When intractable oozing of the vault occurs after vaginal hysterectomy, a suction catheter is placed in the space above the vagina (a Hys-T-Tube is preferred), a large pack is inserted, a catheter is placed in the bladder, and prophylactic antibiotic therapy is instituted. The pack should be removed after 24 hours, the suction catheter after 48 hours or when drainage has ceased, the bladder catheter removed after four days if the patient is afebrile, and the antibiotics discontinued after five days if the patient is afebrile.

When dealing with superficial bleeding from the vagina or vulva, adequate drainage and pressure in the form of a pack or dressing may suffice. The same basic rules apply as for oozing from the vaginal vault. Rarely should it be necessary to open up the operative site to ligate a bleeding vessel after vulvectomy. Adequate suction drainage should prevent such a problem.

While ligation of the hypogastric artery has been necessary on occasion with radical or difficult abdominal surgery, I have never used this technique after radical vulvectomy and lymphadenectomy or after major vaginal surgery. If ligation of the hypogastric artery is deemed necessary, it is best approached via the retroperitoneal space by reopening the inguinal incision in the case of deep lymphadenectomy with vulvectomy. After vaginal hysterectomy, laparotomy is the procedure of choice to determine if the ovarian blood supply has contributed to the bleeding. One or both hypogastric arteries may then be ligated at the junctions with the common iliac artery or at the junction of the anterior and posterior trunks. Ligation of this artery controls hemorrhage by reducing the pulse pressure at the bleeding site.

INJURY

A selective review of the literature for vaginal hysterectomy with or without repair reveals the following incidence of injury: bladder, 24 in 8,999 cases (0.3 per cent); rectum, eight in 9,965 cases (0.1 per cent);

and ureter, six in 14,200 cases (0.04 per cent). Injury of the urethra is documented by Gray's report (1966) of 810 patients with one injury noted at the time of operation and seven patients with postoperative urethrovaginal fistulas.

The surgeon should be alert to any possible injury at the time of operation, for repair at that time usually prevents postoperative fistula. For bladder and rectal injuries the same technique applies as for repair of the simple fistula — initial closure with a continuous 2–0 or 3–0 chromic catgut submucosal suture, followed by one or two layers of reinforcing plicating sutures, and covered by healthy vaginal mucosa. Adequate catheter drainage of the bladder for 10 to 14 days is appropriate for the bladder injury. In the instance of a small rectal injury, prolongation of intravenous fluids and avoidance of constipation should suffice. With a large rectal injury or much tissue destruction, it would be wise to perform a colostomy.

Postoperative leakage of urine or feces may occur hours, days, or weeks after operation and be the first sign of injury. When a urinary fistula is suspected, a tampon may be inserted into the vagina, and phenazopyridine hydrochloride (Pyridium), 200 mg orally, is prescribed; the orange urine will discolor the tip of the tampon. A No. 18 5 cc Foley catheter is inserted and connected to low intermittent suction. Control of the drainage confirms the diagnosis of a vesicovaginal fistula. The catheter should be left in place for six weeks, and suction can be replaced by straight tube drainage after one week. Antibiotics may be given for one week. Conjugated estrogen, 1.25 mg daily for six weeks, may enhance healing in the absence of ovarian function. Surgical management of vesicovaginal fistula will be discussed later.

If the rectal injury is noted immediately after operation, simple repair may be carried out. Otherwise, a period of observation is in order to see if spontaneous closure will occur. If spontaneous healing does not ensue, one of two management programs is recommended. For the small fistula, four to six months should elapse before performing a simple repair. For the large fistula, a colostomy is performed, after four to six months the fistula is repaired, and then after another three months the colostomy is closed.

In contrast to bladder and rectal injury, damage to the ureter usually appears in the form of flank pain, postoperative fever, leakage of urine, or all three beginning from the 3rd to the 21st day after operation. When the injury is noted at operation, a Silastic catheter is threaded into the ureter extending from above the injury to the bladder. If the ureter has been crushed by a clamp with no visible defect, a slit is made above the site of injury for insertion of the catheter, and adequate suction drainage is provided at the site of injury via another Silastic catheter. Delayed leakage of fluid from the vagina can be identified as urine by the use of the vaginal tampon and phenazopyridine hydrochloride. Lack of control by a Foley catheter suggests a ureteral source for the urine. Intravenous pyelography followed by cystoscopy and the intravenous injection of indigo carmine will identify the site of the injury. At the time of cystoscopy, an attempt should be made to pass a ureteral catheter for drainage for 10 days. If the catheter cannot be passed and the kidney continues to function via the ureterovaginal fistula, nephrostomy is not needed. Observe the patient for six weeks before exploration for a ureteroureteral anastomosis or for implantation of the ureter into the bladder. Thompson (1977) has been able to perform an anastomosis via the vagina; however, most surgeons may be more competent and comfortable with the transabdominal approach. The work of Zinman and associates (1978) presents a good discussion of the varied management of ureteral injury with the latter approach.

Focal urethral injury responds to simple closure. Extensive injury requires reconstruction of a urethra and special reinforcement of the vesicourethral angle, as presented elsewhere in this text.

To avoid injury to the femoral nerve during inguinal lymphadenectomy, care must be taken in the region of the femoral canal, especially in the presence of fixed nodes with metastatic cancer. Also, care must be taken in mobilizing the medial border of the sartorius muscle if this is to be transplanted over the femoral canal. Once transected, the femoral nerve can be restored by a direct reconnection or with a nerve graft at the time of operation or later; a neurosurgeon should be consulted.

PELVIC INFECTION

Fortunately, serious infections are rare after surgery of the vulva and vagina. Oozing of blood at the operative site, combined with an increase in bacteria in the genital area, predisposes to wound infections, vaginal cuff infections, pelvic cellulitis, pelvic abscesses, and pelvic thrombophlebitis. In mild form, most such infections manifest themselves as febrile morbidity, which ranges from 30 to 50 per cent in the case of vaginal hysterectomy.

Much attention has been focused on febrile morbidity in the past decade. Prior to this era the main effort was directed to the importance of physical and antiseptic cleansing of the genital area, together with adequate hemostasis. Thomsen (1976) was the first to report marked reduction in febrile morbidity by using prophylactic antibiotics — from 63 to 3 per cent after vaginal hysterectomy with and without repair. Many reports have supported Thomsen's initial observations. Swartz (1979) has shown a significant reduction in febrile morbidity, patient discomfort, postoperative medications, and financial cost when a suction catheter is employed above the vaginal cuff or when prophylactic antibiotics are used or both. Suction catheters and antibiotics have been used for many years with vulvectomy and lymphadenectomy. Osborne and associates (1979) have reduced morbidity by performing hot conization of the cervix before vaginal hysterectomy.

Many varied antibiotic programs have been effective. Our group has favored sodium cephalothin, using 1 gm in 100 cc of intravenous fluid at the beginning of operation, and repeating this dose every six hours until the first or second postoperative day. Cephalexin monohydrate, 500 mg, has been given orally for 48 hours after discontinuing intravenous fluids. An alternative prophylactic antibiotic program consists of tetracycline, 100 mg given intramuscularly every eight hours for one to two days, followed by 500 mg orally every six hours. Recent reports indicate that this additional use of oral antibiotics is unnecessary. We have used the suction catheter selectively in the presence of excessive oozing at or above the vaginal cuff. To the contrary, Swartz (1979) advocated the routine use of the suction catheter with the addition of antibiotics in the premenopausal patient.

The rare serious pelvic infection usually responds to a triple antibiotic program utilizing ampicillin, 500 to 1,000 mg intravenously every six hours; gentamicin sulfate (Garamycin), 60 to 80 mg intravenously or intramuscularly every eight hours; and clindamycin phosphate (Cleocin), 600 mg intravenously every six to eight hours. Schwarz (1978) favors a sequential approach, initiating antibiotic therapy first with penicillin or ampicillin, adding an aminoglycoside (gentamicin) if there is no response, and finally adding clindamycin as necessary or if *Bacteroides fragilis* is suspected. If the patient is allergic to penicillin, a cephalosporin (approximately 5 per cent of penicillin-sensitive patients will have an allergic reaction) and gentamicin or clindamycin and gentamicin may be employed with the use of chloramphenicol (Chloromycetin) in reserve. The desired improvement may not result if a large abscess or pelvic thrombophlebitis is present. In the former instance a tender mass is palpable. If spontaneous drainage does not occur, surgical drainage may be necessary, preferably through the midvaginal apex into a well-defined fluctuant mass; rarely, abdominal exploration, drainage, and even removal of infected tubes and ovaries may be necessary. In the case of thrombophlebitis, a patient with intractable fever and chills will usually respond to heparin within two days. The heparin and antibiotics should be continued for one week.

URINARY TRACT INFECTION

Although it poses no immediate threat to life, urinary tract infection is nevertheless the most frequent infection associated with surgery of the vulva and vagina. This results mainly from the frequent use of the indwelling bladder catheter, but I noted an 18 per cent incidence of such infections after vaginal hysterectomy when repair was not performed and when an indwelling catheter was not used.

Urinary tract infections can be reduced by employing strict sterile technique when inserting a catheter, by using a closed drainage system, and by irrigating the catheter only when absolutely necessary. A catheter should not remain in any longer than necessary, for the potential for infection increases with the duration of the indwelling catheter. When a catheter is to remain in over 24 hours, I prefer a suprapubic Silastic catheter (No. 12 Cystocath). This does not eliminate the threat of infection but does enhance patient comfort and permits better control when the patient begins to void. On the other hand, use of the suprapubic Silastic catheter requires more attention to avoid twisting, kinking, tearing, and obstruction of the lumen. Also, prolapse of the catheter via the urethra may occur with voiding and require cutting of the catheter flush with the urethra with a sterile scissors and withdrawing it into the bladder.

Kass (1957), a world authority on bacteriuria and urinary tract infections, reported the incidence of significant bacteriuria 23 years ago: 6 per cent of 337 female outpatients in the medical service, 18 per cent of women with diabetes, 23 per cent of women with cystocele, 98 per cent of patients with indwelling catheters for 96 hours, and 2 per cent of patients without previous bacteriuria who underwent a single catheterization. When these facts are translated into management of our patients, it would seem wise to send all initial catheter specimens from surgery for routine culture and sensitivity studies. Before removal of an indwelling catheter that has been in place more than 48 hours, a specimen should be sent for culture and sensitivity tests. If any urinary symptom or any poorly defined disease is evident, the urine should be sent for culture and sensitivity studies. Appropriate therapy should be initiated and continued for 10 days; liberal intake of fluids should be encouraged. Nitrofurantoin, 100 mg by mouth every eight hours, may be started while waiting for the culture results. A follow-up culture and sensitivity study should be obtained during a return office visit.

PROLAPSE OF FALLOPIAN TUBE

Prolapse of the fallopian tube through the vaginal cuff may be mistaken for granulation tissue. It can be avoided by eliminating the pursestring closure of the peritoneum and by closing the vaginal cuff.

REMOTE COMPLICATIONS

In a long-term follow-up study of 1,000 patients who had had vaginal hysterectomies, I found that granulation tissue, dyspareunia, stress incontinence of urine, and pronounced recurrent vaginal relaxation occurred in 9, 4, 2, and 1 per cent of patients respectively. Dyspareunia may be reduced by avoiding an overzealous repair. Development of stress incontinence after vaginal repair might be avoided by leaving a gap between the vesicourethral angle and the cystocele repair and by not "overrepairing" the cystocele. The postoperative enterocele may be eliminated if it is recognized and corrected at the time of the initial operation. However, overall it is better to "underrepair" than to "overrepair."

MORTALITY

Among studies of 20,926 patients with vaginal hysterectomies surveyed by me, 28 deaths occurred for an incidence of 0.13 per cent. The cause of death is not noted in most reports. In seven patients the cause was stated as pulmonary embolism in three (one not confirmed by autopsy), peritonitis in two, cerebral aneurysm in one, and ovarian carcinoma in one. Death rates for radical vulvectomy and lymphadenectomy ranged up to 5 per cent, mainly from pulmonary embolism. Whether selective use of prophylactic subcutaneous heparin will reduce deaths from pulmonary embolism remains to be seen.

CONCLUSION

By following the basic principles outlined in this text, the reader will be better able to perform the vast majority of procedures for minor and major surgery of the vulva and vagina. For the most part, this book presents a simple, commonsense approach to benign and malignant problems. Since wide variation exists in the manifestation of disease, the surgeon should be at liberty to alter the scope of the procedure, the technique, and the type and strength of suture material employed, yet at the same time he or she should adhere to the basic concepts presented.

A final brief comment must be made concerning unnecessary surgery, for this issue is very complex and very important. Since most surgical procedures included in this book deal with improving the quality of life for the patient, it might be helpful for the patient herself to render an opinion as to whether attempted surgical relief of her problem is worth the risk, the discomfort, and the expense. In equivocal situations a second professional opinion may correct misrepresentation of symptoms by the patient or misinterpretation of such symptoms by the physician. We must all be wary of the emotionally unstable patient, especially when dealing with vague pelvic pain, menstrual symptoms, and symptoms of pelvic relaxation. It is not an easy task, for we sometimes tend to underrespond to organic disease or to overrespond to hysteria.

Having been a student of vulvovaginal surgery for the past 25 years, I enjoy reviewing surgical textbooks and find that many suggestions by the authors can be put to practical use. We, the surgical and artistic authors, hope and trust that some of our suggested technical approaches will enhance your daily surgical practice and the welfare of your patients.

Minor Vulvovaginal Surgery

BIOPSY OF THE VULVA

Comments. Biopsy of the vulva is an office procedure, except when a large area of abnormal tissue must be excised or when many biopsy specimens must be taken. Staining the vulva with toluidine blue is of debatable merit and is not done. A biopsy should be performed on any questionable area of the vulva. A small representative sample of an obvious lesion, such as a wart, should be taken before chemical or other fulguration.

Technique for Office Biopsy. Lidocaine hydrochloride 1 per cent (Xylocaine) is injected beneath and around the lesion through a single site using a No. 25 needle. After several minutes have elapsed, a 4 mm disposable Baker's biopsy punch is rotated through the full thickness of the skin (Fig. 1 *A* and *B*); a fine forceps is used to elevate the small circular piece of tissue, and fine scissors free the biopsy specimen from the subcutaneous tissue (Fig. 1 *C*). The biopsy site is lightly cauterized with a portable electrocautery point. On rare occasions, a figure-of-eight fine polyglycolic acid (Davis & Geck CE4 Dexon 3–0) or nylon suture with a small cutting needle is required.

Technique for Hospital Biopsy. The lesion is circumscribed to a depth of several millimeters. Bleeding vessels are clamped and ligated with 3–0 chromic catgut or polyglycolic acid sutures. No subcutaneous closing sutures are used, but the skin is approximated with simple or figure-of-eight Tevdek 2–0 sutures. These sutures may be removed in the office in five to ten days; the longer time is preferred if there is any tension on the suture line.

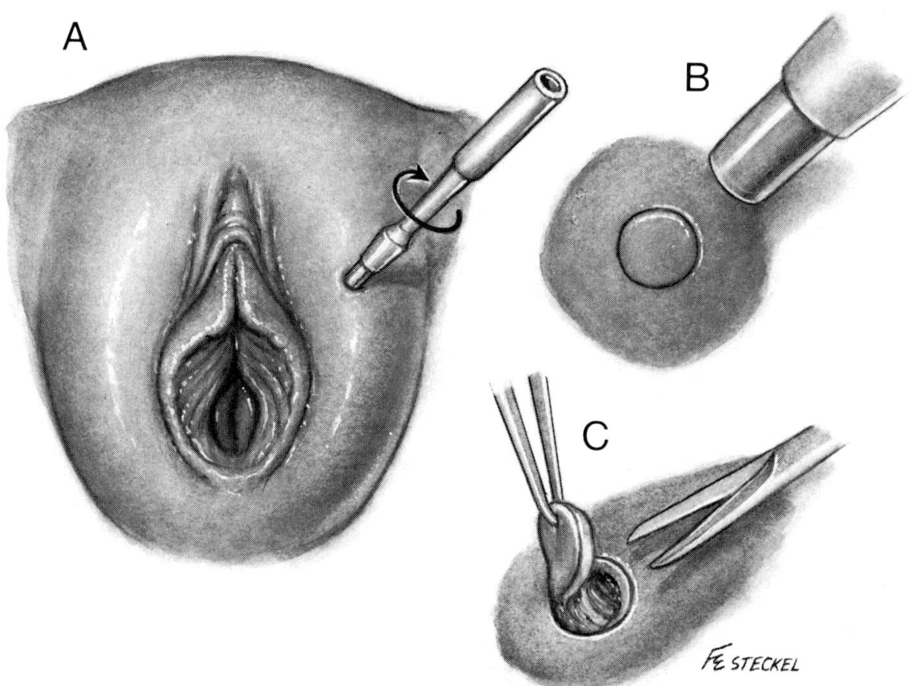

Figure 1. *A* through *C*, Office biopsy of vulva using a round, sharp, and disposable 4 mm biopsy punch.

ALCOHOL INJECTION OF THE VULVA

Comments. Alcohol injection is a rare procedure used for intractable pruritus vulvae in the absence of any demonstrable disease and in the absence of any response to observation and conservative measures. General anesthesia is required.

Technique. After the genital area is routinely prepared and draped, indigo carmine or another dye is used to draw vertical and horizontal lines over the vulva and adjacent skin, demarcating 1 cm squares of skin.

At each junction of the lines or for each square centimeter of skin, 0.1 cc of 95 per cent alcohol is injected subcutaneously by tuberculin syringe. After the injections, the skin is massaged gently to improve the distribution of alcohol in the subcutaneous fat. Do not inject the alcohol intradermally, and do not inject the alcohol into the adjacent mucosa.

Postoperative Considerations. Adequate pain medication must be prescribed, for the patient may have a combination of discomfort and numbness in the genital area. Inspection of the skin on the following day may show diffuse erythema and mild edema. The patient should have no difficulty voiding and should be ready for discharge from the hospital within 24 hours.

BIOPSY OF THE CERVIX

Comments. Biopsy of the cervix is usually performed in the office. Biopsy specimens should be taken of all abnormal areas; if colposcopy is available, it should be used to delineate precisely the more suspicious points for biopsy. If the cervix appears normal macroscopically but the Papanicolaou test reveals suspicious cells, the cervical canal should be curetted (see section on curettage). Colposcopic examination should be performed if available, the cervix and upper vagina should be stained with a concentrated Schiller's solution (1 gm iodine, 2 gm potassium iodide, 300 cc water), and biopsy specimens should be taken of any questionable area on the ectocervix. In summary, any abnormal area, any area not stained with Schiller's solution, and any suspicious colposcopic finding should be biopsied, taking multiple biopsy specimens as necessary.

Technique. A Wittner cervical biopsy punch (curved or straight) or an Eppendorfer cervical biopsy forceps is used, with its teeth placed at the base of the biopsy site, and a biopsy specimen is taken decisively and quickly. Occasionally it is necessary to hold the cervix steady with an iris hook or with a tenaculum (Fig. 2). After the biopsy samples are taken, a tampon is opened, placed against the cervix, and reinforced with a second tampon if necessary. The patient is allowed to rest on the examining table for five minutes to make certain that the bleeding is controlled. If bleeding continues, supplementary cautery or a figure-of-eight suture (Davis & Geck CE4 Dexon 3–0 or Ethicon N878) is applied. The needle holder is placed at the middle of the suture needle to avoid breaking the needle in the hard tissue of the cervix. It is prudent to have a long, narrow needle holder in the office for such a procedure.

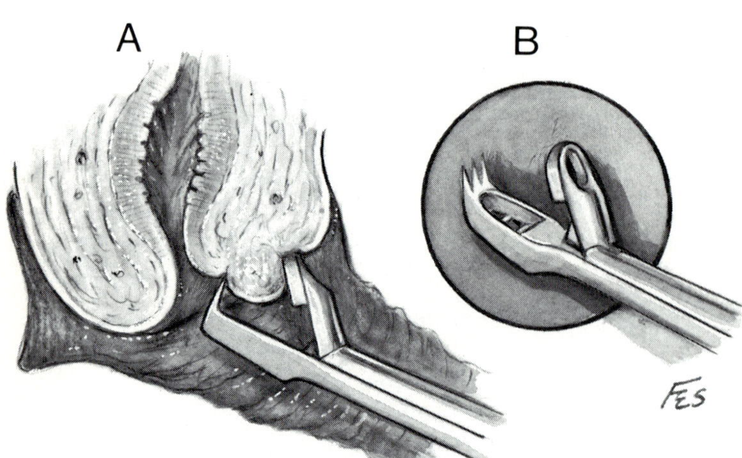

Figure 2. *A* and *B,* Biopsy of cervix with straight Wittner biopsy punch.

REMOVAL OF A CERVICAL POLYP

Comments. A true cervical polyp is rarely malignant. On the other hand, carcinoma of the cervix and endometrium may present as a polypoid lesion in the cervical canal. A polyp also may be the source of present or future abnormal bleeding. Large polyps or those with wide stalks are best removed in the hospital, where the bleeding operative site may be visualized and sutured.

Technique. To preserve the polyp for pathologic examination, avoid crushing the tissue with a clamp. It is preferable to use a cervical biopsy forceps to hold the polyp and to twist the polyp with multiple rotations until it can be removed with ease.

CURETTAGE OF THE ENDOCERVIX

Comments. Curettage may be performed in the office or as the initial part of a dilatation and curettage procedure (which will be discussed later). It is indicated in the presence of abnormal bleeding of unknown origin and when results of a Papanicolaou test are questionable, suspicious, or positive.

Technique. The cervix may or may not have to be held in place by a tenaculum on the anterior lip. The cervical canal is thoroughly scraped for a distance of 3 cm with a Kevorkian-Younge endocervical biopsy curet (Fig. 3). A small amount of bloody mucus is usually obtained, placed on a Telfa pad or on a piece of nonabsorbing paper, and then placed in a fixative solution. A toothpick is helpful in removing the material from the curet.

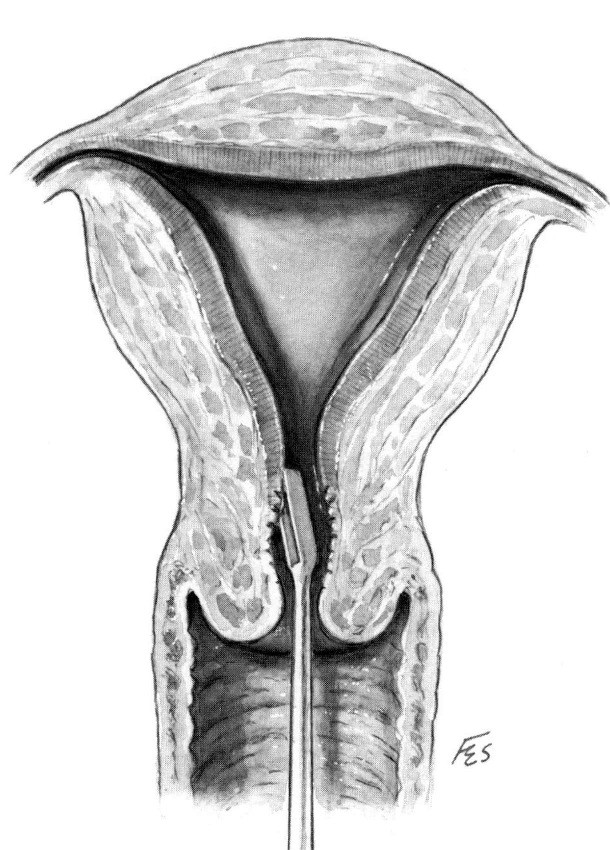

Figure 3. Endocervical curettage with Kevorkian-Younge curet.

BIOPSY OF THE ENDOMETRIUM

Comments. Biopsy of the endometrium is performed in the office in order to obtain a sample of endometrium for evaluation of infertility or amenorrhea when pregnancy is not suspected. The specimen is obtained at the beginning of menstruation or in the premenstrual phase of the cycle when assessing infertility. A premenstrual serum progesterone determination also may be used to confirm ovulation.

Technique. The apprehensive patient may be given 1 grain of codeine and two aspirin tablets by mouth 15 minutes before the procedure. An examination is performed to ascertain the position of the uterus. A regular clean speculum is inserted, and the cervix is cleansed twice with povidone-iodine solution. A sterile, single-toothed tenaculum is placed on the anterior lip of the cervix, and a sterile, standard Meigs endometrial biopsy curet (9.5 inch or 24.13 cm) is inserted for the full length of the uterine cavity and scraped along the endometrium as it is withdrawn (Fig. 4). If satisfactory contact is not felt, the instrument should be turned over and the same maneuver repeated. If this standard instrument will not pass the cervix, then a microcuret may be used (see next section). The patient will experience pelvic cramps, which gradually subside after the procedure. Slight bleeding may persist for several days.

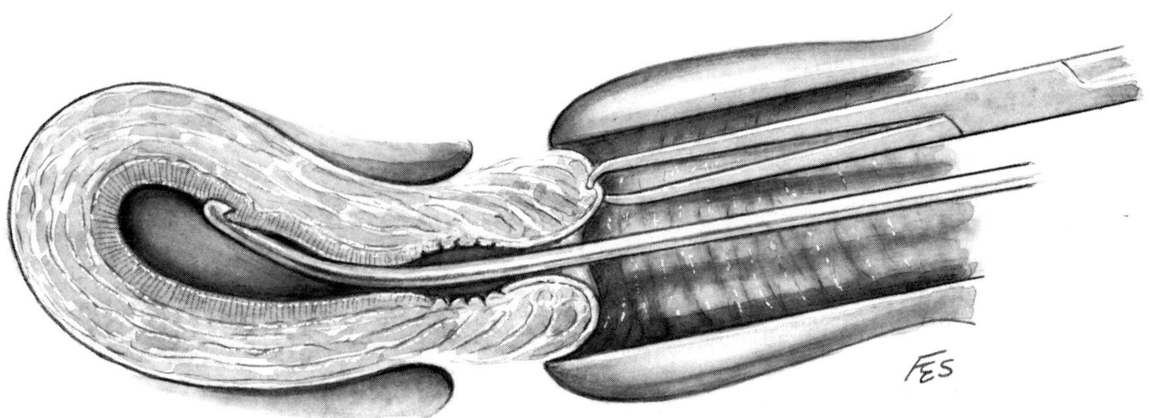

Figure 4.   Simple endometrial biopsy with Meigs endometrial biopsy curet.

ASPIRATION OF THE UTERINE CAVITY

Comments. Aspiration, an office procedure, is performed when multiple samples of the endometrium are desired but borderline indication exists for hospital curettage and when rapid confirmation of uterine malignancy is desired.

Technique. The preparation is the same as that used for the standard endometrial biopsy. A sterile Randall endometrial biopsy suction curet (3 mm, Luer hub, 9.25 inch or 23.50 cm) is used with a 20 cm syringe attached. The nurse steadies the tenaculum, and the patient is advised that she will have a "sick crampy discomfort" that will gradually fade away after the one-minute procedure. The operator aspirates with the syringe as the curet is scraped and rotated over one side of the uterine cavity (Fig. 5); the same maneuver is then applied to the opposite side. Commercial suction devices may be used but are not necessary.

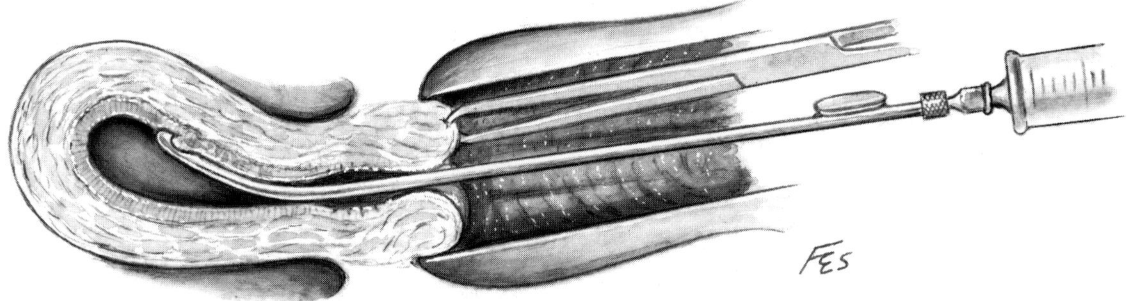

Figure 5.　Office endometrial aspiration with Randall 3 mm suction curet.

DILATATION AND CURETTAGE

Comments. In contrast to the office procedure described, it is best to perform dilatation and curettage in the hospital or in a clinic immediately adjacent to the hospital so that emergency resuscitation measures are available. This procedure is indicated for any unexplained abnormal bleeding of uterine origin and may improve functional or dysfunctional bleeding. Suction evacuation of the uterus followed by curettage is used to interrupt early pregnancies of up to 13 weeks' gestation. Although it is not within the purview of this text to discuss abortions at length, the reader is referred to the bibliography regarding the use of Laminaria to permit dilatation of the cervix and extraction of the fetus up to 20 weeks' gestation. Persistent unexplained discharge from the uterus also justifies a diagnostic curettage. When this procedure is considered, it is also important to remember that abnormal bleeding may be present with a threatened miscarriage, and interruption or termination of a desired pregnancy must be avoided. Although the procedure may be performed under a combination of sedation and hypnosis or under local, spinal, or general anesthesia, we usually have used general anesthesia because it permits the most satisfactory manual examination.

A thorough examination under anesthesia should, of course, precede any dilatation and curettage, for abnormal bleeding not only may reflect problems within the uterine cavity but also may be associated with lesions in the cervix ·and vagina and with adnexal disease, such as ectopic pregnancy, malignancy of the tube, benign cysts and tumors of the ovaries, and malignant tumors of the ovaries.

Technique. In addition to routine preparation and draping, intravenous antibiotics should be given with the termination of a septic abortion (see section on preoperative evaluation and care). If early pregnancy exists, intramuscular oxytocin (Pitocin), 10 units, should be administered. The anterior lip of the cervix is grasped with a tenaculum. If local anesthesia is used, 1 per cent lidocaine, 5 cc, is injected 1 cm out from the external cervical os, distributing the anesthetic from a depth of 2 or 3 cm parallel to the cervical canal. Curettage of the endocervical canal is carried out (see section on curettage). The uterus is gently sounded with a uterine sound, and the depth of the uterus in centimeters is carefully noted. The cervix is dilated with Hank or Hegar dilators. If malignancy is suspected, it is best to dilate the cervix only to the degree necessary to allow the introduction of polyp forceps (Randall kidney stone forceps, quarter curved) and a Meigs serrated uterine curet (10 inch or 25.4 cm). However, if pregnancy is to be terminated, it is better to dilate the cervix as much as possible. Overzealous curettage in the presence of malignancy is to be avoided; just enough tissue should be obtained to permit frozen section examination. The serrated curet is introduced to the full depth of the uterus, rotated around the circumference of the uterine cavity, and scraped against the endometrium (Fig. 6). The polyp forceps is then used to explore the uterus (Fig. 7). In the case of curettage for dysfunctional bleeding, a sharp curet is used to scrape the entire circumference of the uterine cavity repeatedly. If sepsis or tuberculosis is suspected, specimens for culture of aerobic and anaerobic organisms and of tubercle bacilli should be obtained. When an early pregnancy is being terminated, a suction cannula with a diameter appropriate for the cervical canal should be inserted, a maximum vacuum obtained, and the cannula rotated until the collection tubing contains only frothy, blood-tinged fluid (Fig. 8). The uterine cavity is curetted in a routine manner, and an open sponge is inserted and rotated within the uterine cavity to make certain that all tissue has been removed.

Postoperative Considerations. Any vaginal sponge or pack should be removed in the recovery room and replaced with pads as necessary. An antibiotic program should be begun if sepsis is apparent or if medical status indicates. If the uterus has been perforated, the patient should be observed closely for 24 to 48 hours. If pregnancy has been terminated and the patient is Rh negative, immune globulin (RhoGAM), 1 cc, should be given intramuscularly. Intravenous fluids may be discontinued when the patient is awake and alert. The bladder should be catheterized only if necessary. Mild pain medications, such as codeine and aspirin, may be given by mouth at four-hour intervals. If bleeding is excessive after an abortion, ergonovine maleate (Ergotrate), 0.2 mg, should be given intramuscularly or by mouth every four hours for six doses provided that the patient does not have hypertension. After four hours the patient may be discharged in the company of a friend or relative, as circumstances and individual considerations permit.

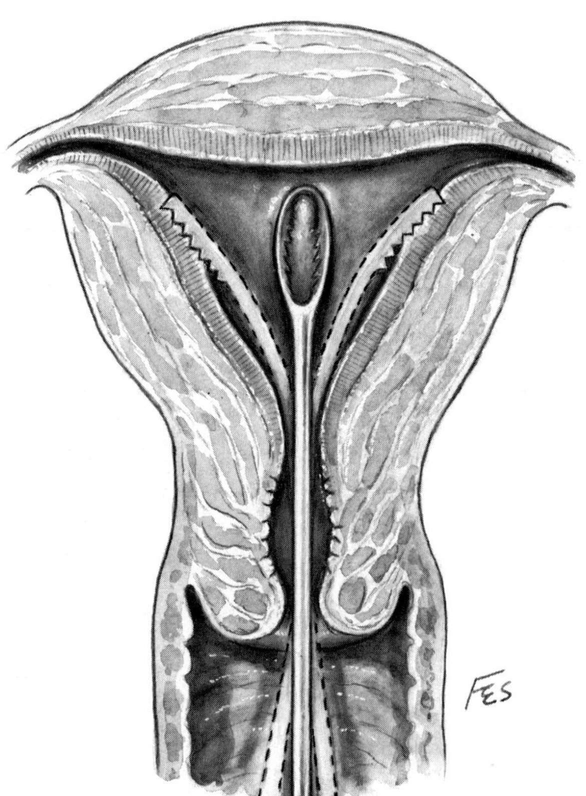

Figure 6. Hospital curettage with Meigs serrated uterine curet.

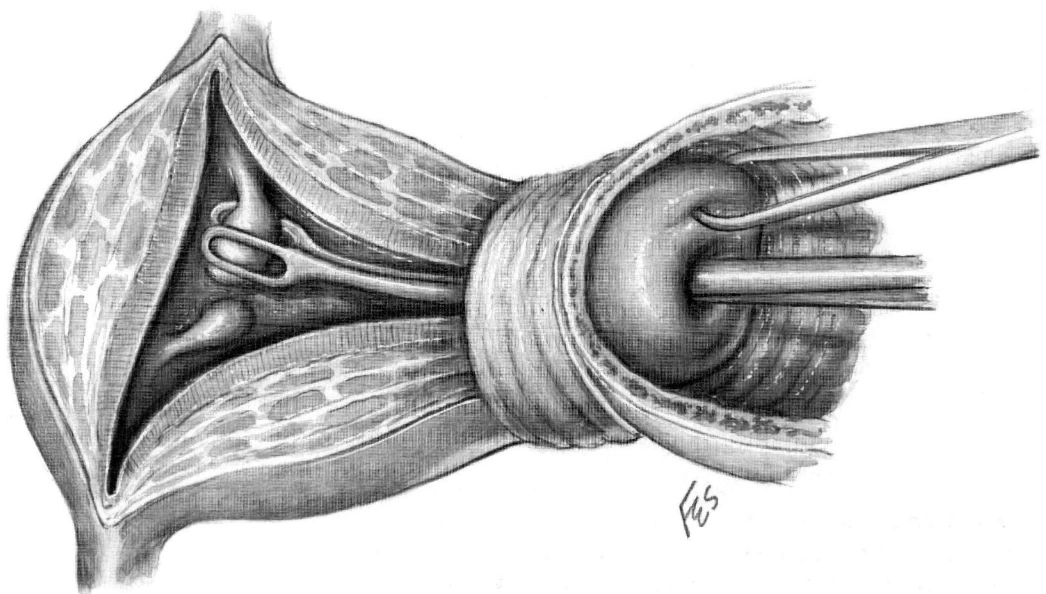

Figure 7. Removal of polyp with slightly curved Randall kidney stone forceps.

Figure 8. Suction curettage for early intrauterine pregnancy.

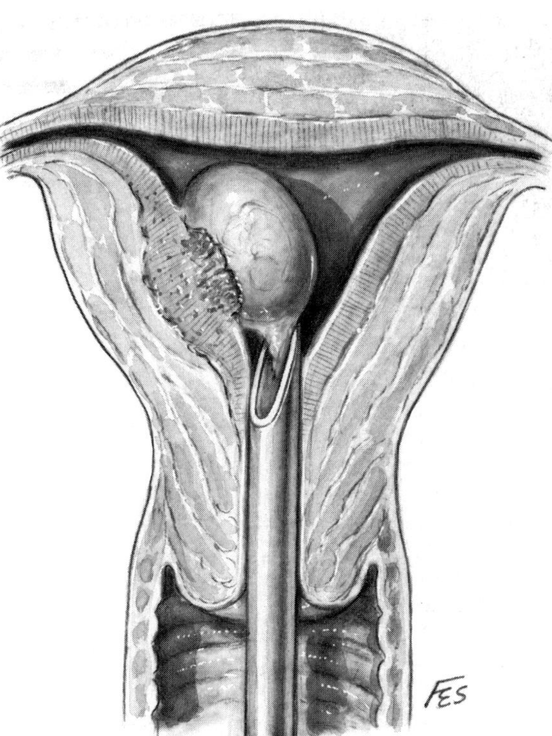

HYSTEROSALPINGOGRAPHY

Comments. Hysterosalpingography is usually performed in the office on a patient in the early phase of the menstrual cycle as part of an infertility evaluation. However, when the procedure is not technically possible or when the patient exhibits undue discomfort, it is performed with a cervical dilatation in the operating room under general anesthesia. Insufflation of the uterus and tubes with carbon dioxide has been discontinued as a diagnostic procedure.

Technique. The patient is prepared and draped as for curettage, the uterus is sounded, and the cervix is partially dilated to permit introduction of a uterine cannula or a No. 8 5 cc Foley catheter (expanding the bulb with air to block the cervical canal). Diatrizoate meglumine and iodipamide meglumine (Sinografin), 10 cc, is instilled via the cannula or catheter, the end of the cannula is closed or the catheter is clamped, and the radiograph or print (Polaroid) is taken within five seconds. Since the radiopaque fluid is thin and water-soluble, it is important to take the radiograph or picture rapidly. On occasion, as in the case of a hydrosalpinx, a second film will be required, using more than 10 cc of Sinografin. However, exertion of too much pressure in the injection of Sinografin should be avoided to prevent possible rupture of an obstructed tube.

Postoperative Considerations. The patient is treated with mild pain medication and discharged from four to 24 hours after the procedure.

CONIZATION OF THE CERVIX

Comments. Conization should be performed when results of a Papanicolaou test are unexplained, suspicious, or positive, and when the patient's condition has remained undiagnosed after colposcopy, Schiller test, biopsy, and endocervical curettage. It should also be done when severe dysplasia and carcinoma in situ are not clearly defined by colposcopy-directed biopsy. Conization may be used for both diagnosis of and therapy for carcinoma in situ in a young woman who has not completed her childbearing. Although this procedure is listed under minor surgery, it may be associated with serious complications, such as operative and postoperative hemorrhage, formation of large hematomas, infections, or abortions. Therefore, this procedure should be used selectively and preferably not at all in the presence of pregnancy or when adequate exposure cannot be obtained. Conization of the cervix should be accomplished soon after completion of the menstrual period. In the presence of poor exposure of the cervix, multiple biopsies may be performed around the cervical os and into the cervical canal as an alternative to conization. The uterus is sounded, the cervix is dilated, and curettage of the uterine cavity is carried out first.

Technique. A deep hemostasis suture is placed at the lateral angle of the cervix near its junction with the vagina, using No. 1 chromic catgut on a large cutting needle (Fig. 9 *A*). These sutures should be held with clamps for exposure. Four tension sutures are placed around the cervical os, using silk for the anterior suture for identification purposes; 1–0 chromic catgut or 2–0 silk may be used on a small Mayo needle (Fig. 9 *B*). All of the tension sutures are placed in one clamp and on tension while a sharp-pointed scalpel (11 ASR stainless steel blade) is used to remove carefully a cone of tissue measuring 1 cm around the external os (or the appropriate width to incorporate colposcopically abnormal areas or areas unstained by the Schiller test) and a depth of 2 cm into the canal (Fig. 10 *A* and *B*). Anterior and posterior Sturmdorf sutures are placed with No. 1 chromic catgut on large cutting needles (Fig. 11 *A*). It is important that the full depth of the conization site be included in the sutures; otherwise serious postoperative bleeding may occur. With a cervical dilator in the canal and pulled to one side, a figure-of-eight No. 1 chromic catgut suture is placed at each lateral angle of the cervix (Fig. 11 *B*). The dilator is removed, and the cervix is observed; additional sutures are placed only as necessary.

Postoperative Considerations. The postoperative considerations are the same as for dilatation and curettage. A vaginal pack is put into place at the operating table and removed two hours after operation. The patient may be discharged on the following day but should be admonished to reduce activity until after her office check-up in two to four weeks. Tampons or douches should not be used and no coitus engaged in during this time.

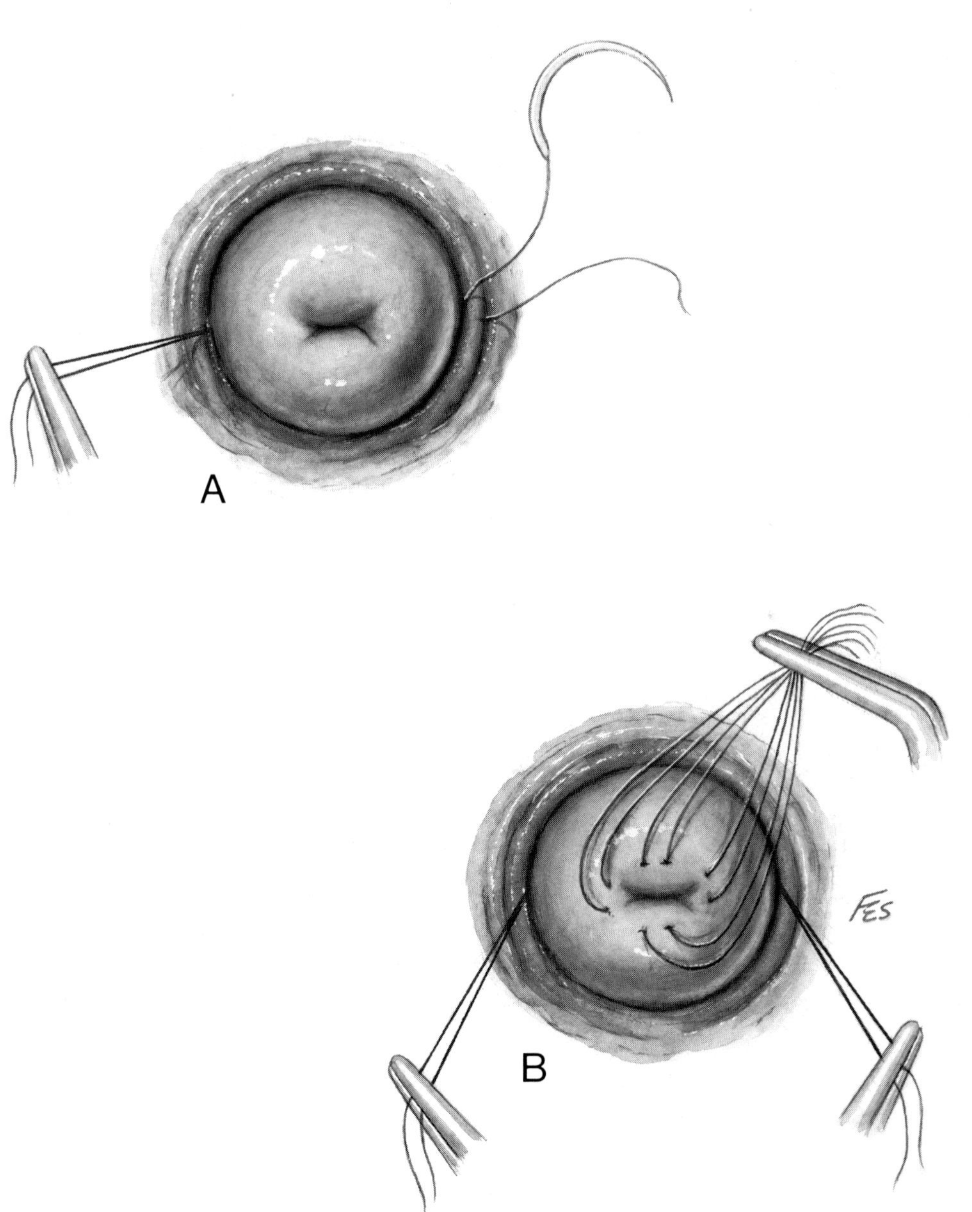

Figure 9. Conization of cervix. *A,* Placement of angled hemostatic sutures followed by *B,* placement of tension sutures around cervical os.

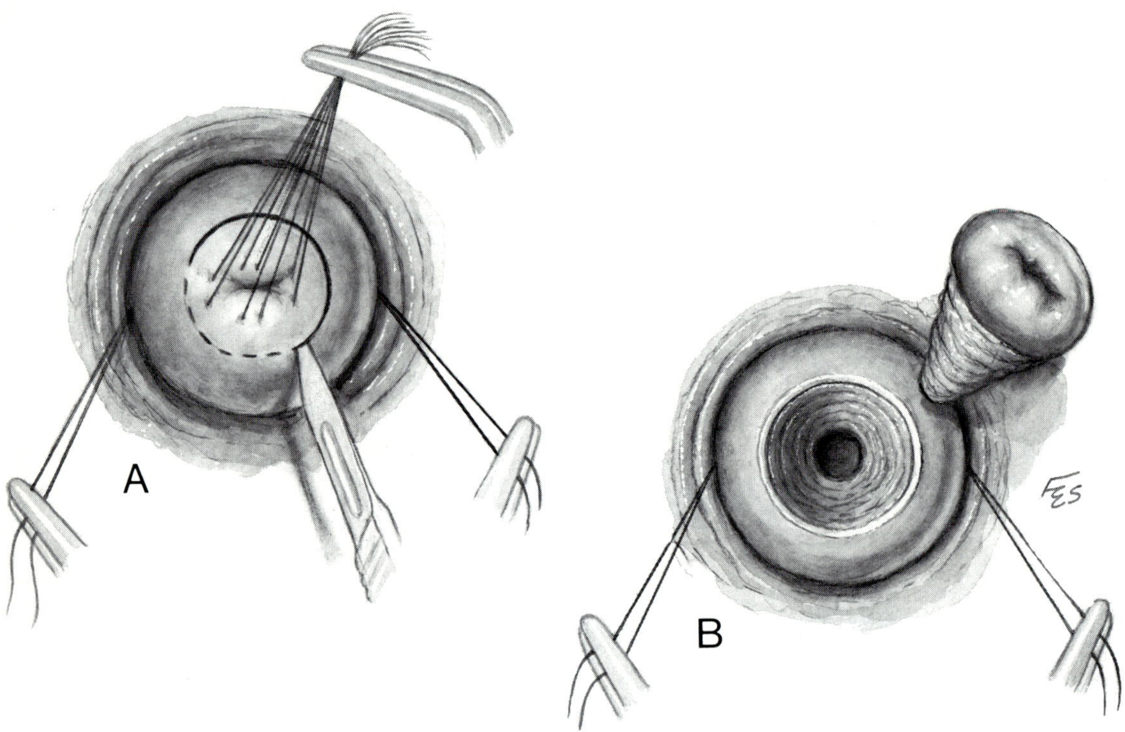

Figure 10. Conization of cervix. *A* and *B,* Excision of cone of cervix.

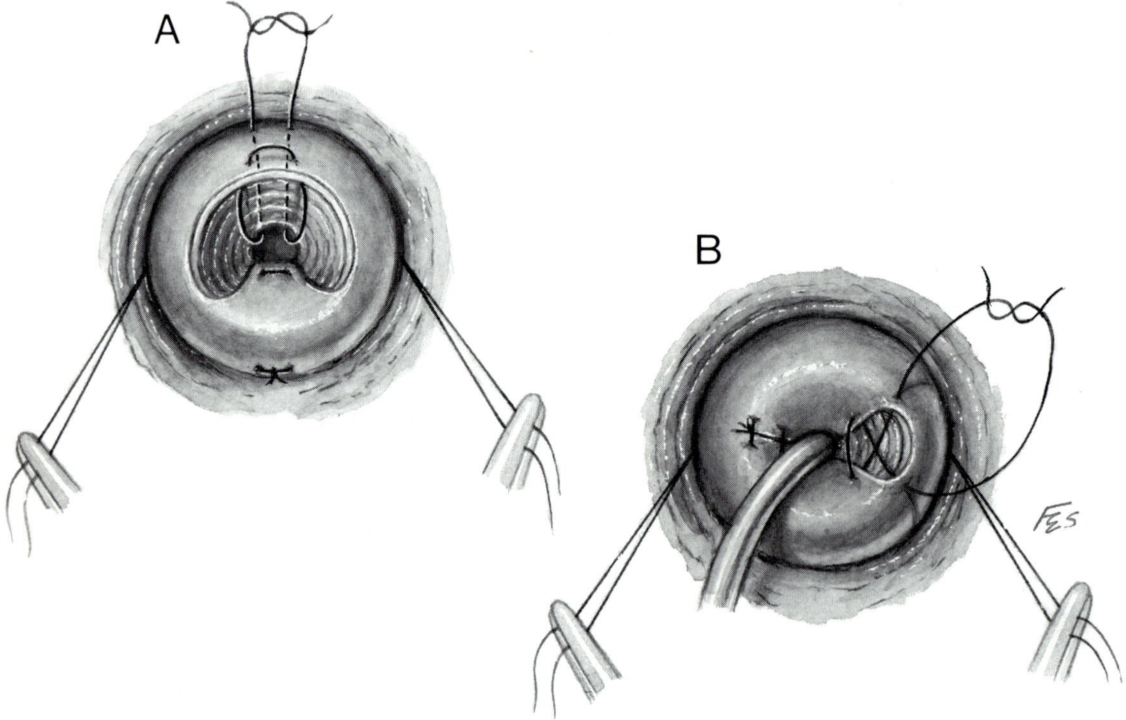

Figure 11. Conization of cervix. *A,* Placement of anterior and posterior Sturmdorf sutures followed by *B,* placement of lateral figure-of-eight sutures.

MARSUPIALIZATION OF
BARTHOLIN CYST OR ABSCESS

Comments. Marsupialization has virtually replaced incision and drainage and excision of the chronically inflamed Bartholin gland in our experience. Only large cysts and abscesses are treated. Because malignancy may occur within the Bartholin gland, it is important to take a biopsy sample of an indurated Bartholin gland. Although hypnosis and local anesthesia have been used, general anesthesia is preferred.

Technique. Saline is injected via a No. 25 needle into the cyst cavity (Fig. 12 *A*). With Allis clamps on the labium to provide exposure, a circle of tissue 1.5 cm in diameter is outlined with the scalpel on the mucosal side of the swelling (Fig. 12 *A*). Once the area of mucosal excision is clear, the bottom half of the cyst is opened (Fig. 12 *B*), and a culture specimen is taken for detection of gonorrhea. Other cultures may be academic because antibiotics are not used. An Allis clamp is used to hold the partially excised circle of tissue upward while interrupted polyglycolic acid sutures (Davis & Geck T5 Dexon 3–0) are placed to attach the mucosa of the gland to the genital mucosa (Fig. 12 *C*). The remainder of the circle of tissue is removed, providing a small circular window into the Bartholin cyst or abscess. The remainder of the mucosa is approximated (Fig. 12 *D*), hemostasis is obtained, and a small iodoform wick is inserted into the cavity of the gland or abscess.

Postoperative Considerations. The postoperative considerations are the same as for dilatation and curettage. The iodoform wick is removed before hospital discharge. The patient is advised to take a warm tub bath once or twice daily until her office check-up in two weeks.

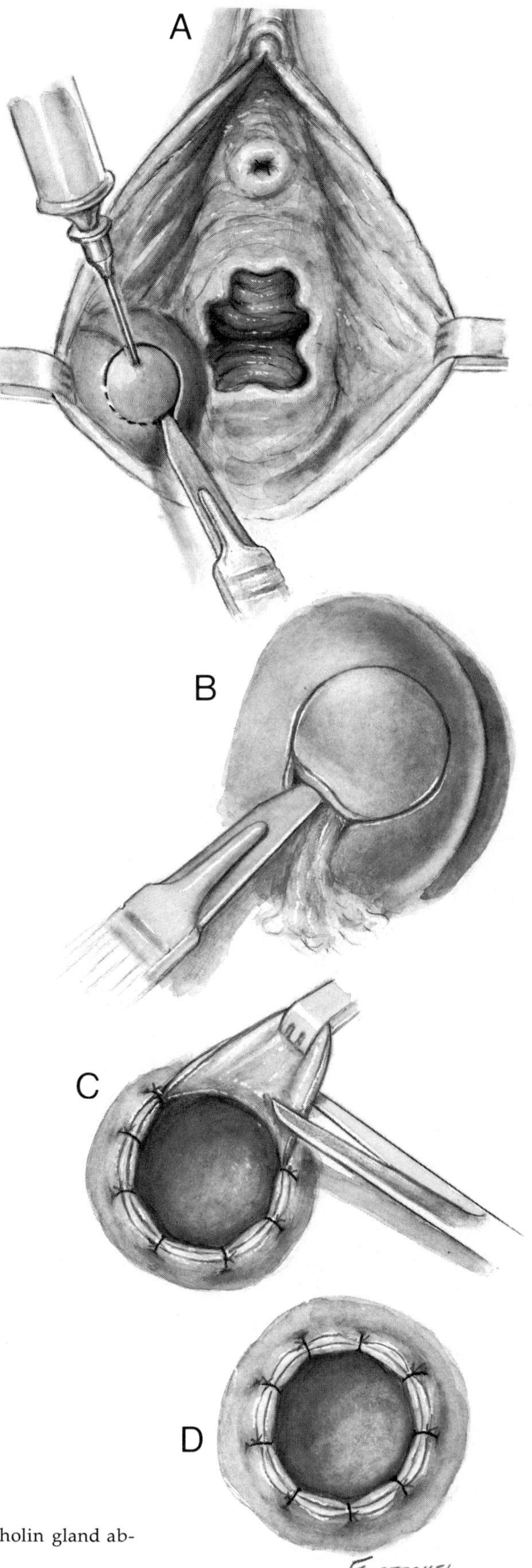

Figure 12. *A* through *D,* Marsupialization of right Bartholin gland abscess.

EXCISION OF CHRONIC BARTHOLINITIS

Comments. Excision of chronic bartholinitis has become a rare procedure in our experience. If an abscess is properly drained through marsupialization as described, chronic inflammation should rarely occur.

Technique. Adequate assistance and exposure are necessary (Fig. 13 *A*). Considerable bleeding may be encountered. A superficial incision is made around the area to be excised. With countertension between the surrounding vulva and the indurated Bartholin gland, the thickened, chronically inflamed tissue is circumscribed and excised (Fig. 13 *B*), clamping and ligating the bleeding vessels as they are exposed. No drain is used, but the entire excision site is approximated with simple or figure-of-eight 2–0 or No. 2 Tevdek sutures (Fig. 13 *C*), using the latter large suture if much tissue tension exists. Better approximation of the tissue is obtained if subcutaneous sutures are avoided.

Postoperative Considerations. A suprapubic Silastic catheter (Dow Cystocath No. 12) is inserted into the bladder. A sterile pad is placed over the vulva, and a cold pack is placed against this pad overnight. Antibiotics are not used unless purulent material was encountered during the operation. On the day after operation, the ice pack is discontinued, and on the second day after operation the patient is allowed to void before the catheter is removed. The patient is discharged on the third postoperative day if her condition permits. She is advised to take a warm tub bath twice daily and is seen in one week for removal of sutures.

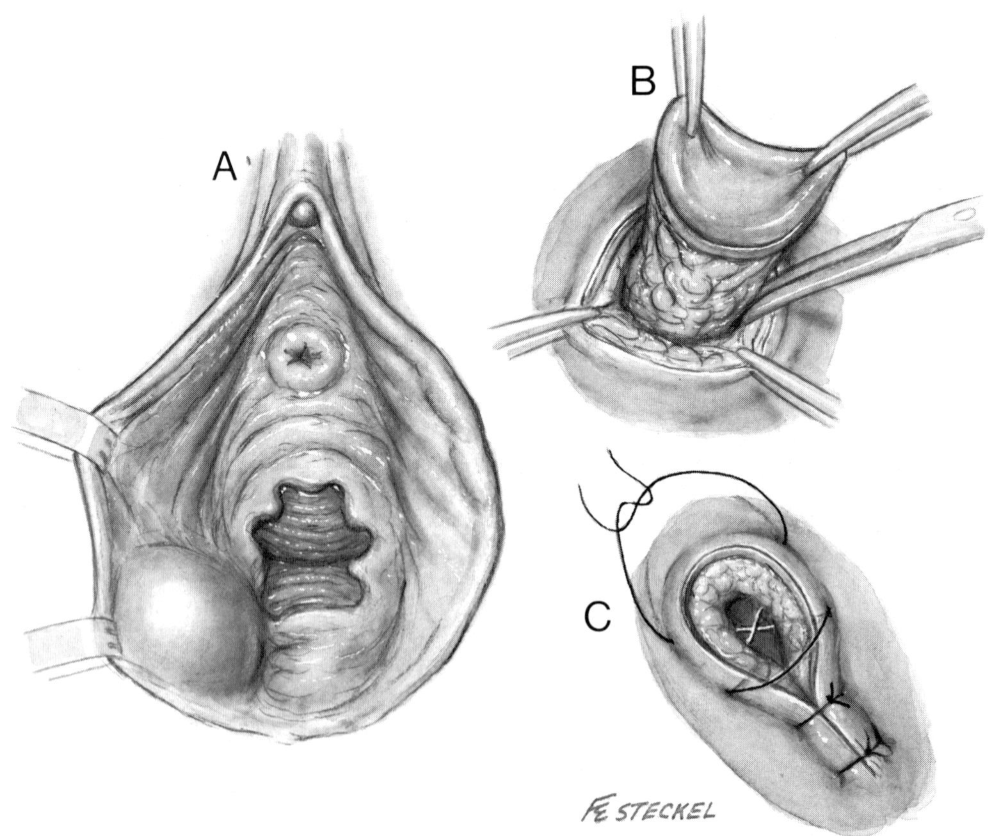

Figure 13.   *A* through *C,* Excision of chronically inflamed right Bartholin gland.

FULGURATION OF WARTS

Comments. A biopsy should be taken to differentiate a condyloma acuminatum, a papilloma, and a carcinoma. Such warts may affect the perineum, the vulva, the adjacent skin, the vaginal mucosa, the cervix, and the anal mucosa. Small, scattered isolated warts are treated by careful application of 25 per cent podophyllin (in tincture of benzoin) or of 50 per cent trichloroacetic acid (aqueous solution) as an office procedure. If repeated applications are ineffective or if the lesions are quite large, fulguration and electrosurgical removal are performed under general anesthesia. We have not found cryosurgical treatment to be helpful.

Technique. With the Bovie electrosurgical machine set between 30 and 40 on coagulation, the small lesions are carefully and precisely fulgurated (Fig. 14 *A*). It is important to use an aqueous solution for preparation and to make certain that the sheet beneath the patient is dry and without any holes or defects. When large lesions are present, the loop cautery is used to remove loops full of the warts (Fig. 14 *B*). At this point, it is sometimes helpful to take a sharp curet and scrape the remainder of the wart-like tissue from its base of attachment to the skin (Fig. 14 *C*), followed by light coagulation of this curetted base. Large lesions have been removed in this manner with a good cosmetic result.

Postoperative Considerations. The postoperative considerations are the same as those for dilatation and curettage. The bladder is not catheterized. The patient is permitted to go home either on the evening of operation or on the day after operation and is advised to take a daily warm tub bath and to avoid any irritation of the treated area by undergarments. The patient may experience moderate discomfort for some days, and adequate pain medication should be prescribed.

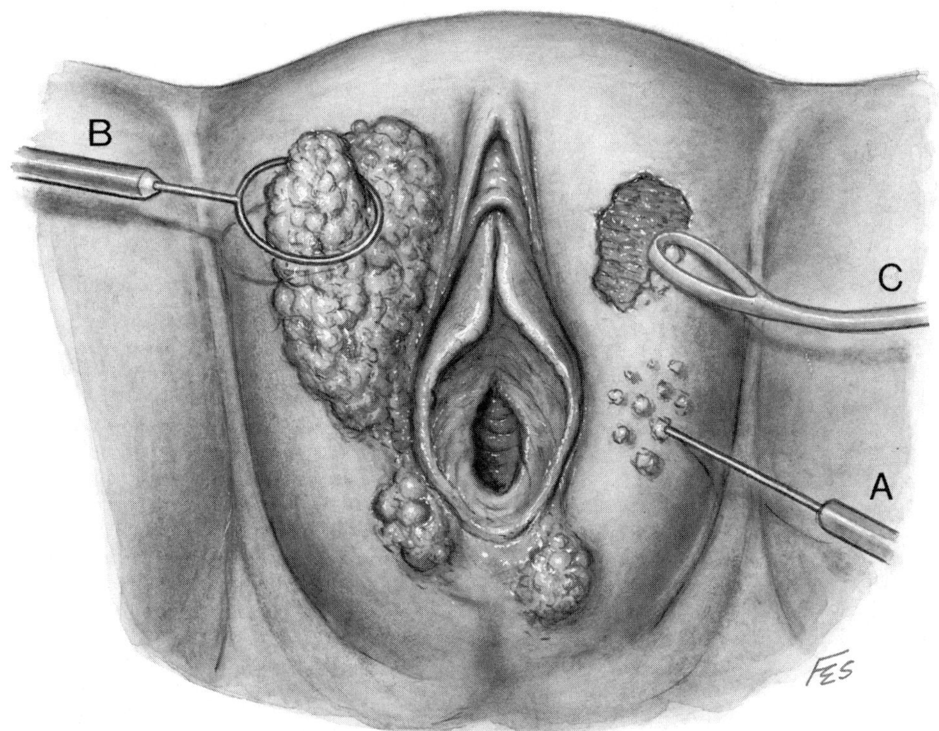

Figure 14. *A* through *C*, Fulguration of condylomata acuminata.

INCISION OF HYMEN

Comments. Rarely, a woman has a stricture of the hymen that requires incision or excision. Prominent hymenal ridges usually stretch with gentle examination and liberal use of a lubricant. In some instances a very thin hymen can be cut quickly at multiple points as an office procedure with or without local anesthesia and sedation. In rare instances in which the hymen is extremely prominent and thickened due to repeated attempts at intercourse or completely occludes the introitus with a secondary hematocolpos, incision and revision in the hospital under general anesthesia are indicated.

Technique. If the hymen is completely intact, a central small opening is made to permit any blood from within the vagina to escape. The hymen is incised at four points, the 10 o'clock, 2 o'clock, 4 o'clock, and 8 o'clock positions (Fig. 15 *A*), and interrupted polyglycolic acid sutures (Davis & Geck T5 Dexon 3–0) are used to close the incisions in a transverse direction (Fig. 15 *B*), making certain that the introitus is not constricted. If the hymen is very redundant, each of the four segments is excised and figure-of-eight sutures are placed around the introitus to approximate the mucosa and to achieve hemostasis.

Postoperative Considerations. A petroleum jelly gauze pack placed in the introitus at operation is removed on the following morning before the patient's discharge. The bladder is catheterized only if necessary. The patient is advised to take a warm tub bath twice daily until her check-up in the office in one week, when the introitus is gently dilated.

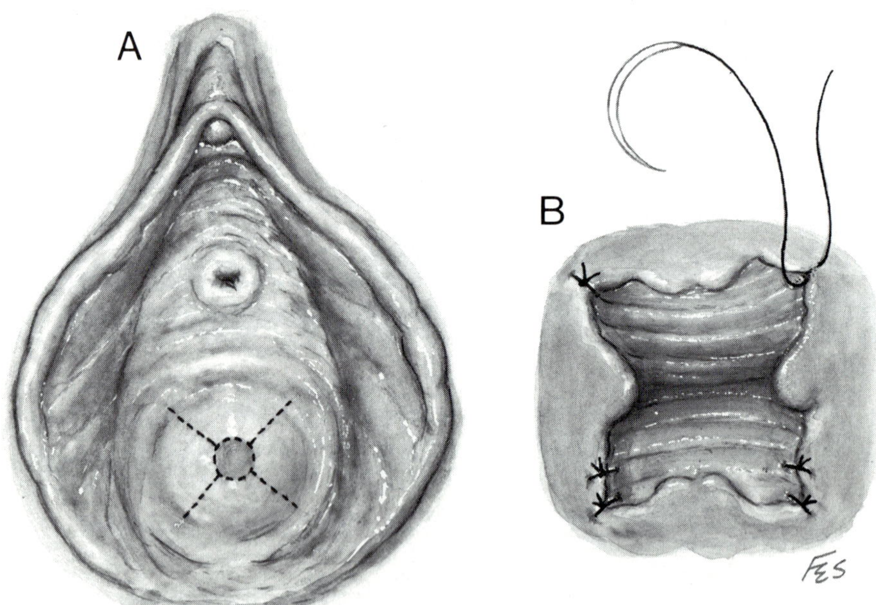

Figure 15. *A* and *B*, Incision of intact hymen.

EXCISION OF VAGINAL CYST OR TUMOR

Comments. Biopsy of small focal suspicious areas in the upper vagina may be performed in the office, usually without any anesthesia, with the Wittner biopsy instrument, as described for the technique for cervical biopsy. For the lower two thirds of the vagina, 1 per cent lidocaine may be injected beneath the biopsy site. Obvious benign Gartner duct cysts and inclusion cysts of the vagina are relegated to periodic check-up visits and are not excised. However, an occasional cyst or nodule in the vaginal wall warrants excision biopsy. If such a lesion is located anteriorly, urologic evaluation should be performed to make certain that it is not a bladder or urethral diverticulum. If a lesion is located on the posterior wall, proctoscopy should be performed to rule out any underlying disease of the rectum. Since the vagina may be the site of metastasis from malignancy, this possibility should be considered when taking the patient's history and examining the patient.

Technique.   Excision of a nodule (Fig. 16 *A*) above the lower part of the vagina may be awkward, and good exposure is important. Allis clamps are used to place the mucosa adjacent to and over the lesion on tension, and a semicircular mucosal incision is made distal to the nodule to allow careful dissection of the base of the lesion from its surrounding attachments (Fig. 16 *B*); this is best done with Metzenbaum scissors (Fig. 16 *C*). The lesion may be detached easily or may require the removal of the mucosa overlying it. The mucosal defect is closed in a transverse direction with interrupted simple or figure-of-eight 3–0 chromic catgut or polyglycolic acid sutures (Fig. 16 *D*).

Postoperative Considerations.   Postoperative considerations are the same as for dilatation and curettage. No pack is used. The bladder is catheterized only as necessary. The patient is advised to insert nothing into the vagina until after her check-up visit in one month. The patient may be discharged as soon as four hours after operation.

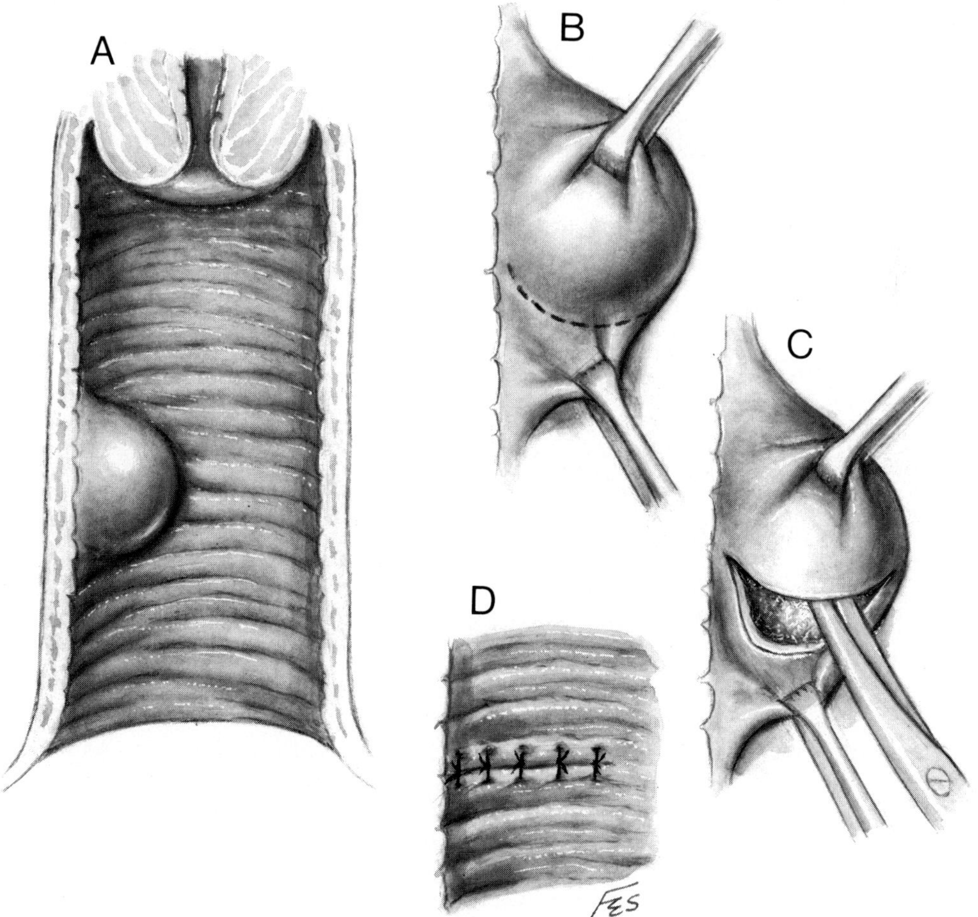

Figure 16.   *A* through *D*, Excision of vaginal cyst.

CULDOSCOPY

Comments. Both culdoscopy and laparoscopy are, for the most part, diagnostic tools employed as a preferred alternative to exploratory laparotomy. Limited operative procedures (biopsy, lysis of adhesions, fulgurations, Silastic banding of tubes) may be done through the culdoscope and laparoscope. Laparoscopy has replaced culdoscopy almost entirely, for the laparoscope provides better visualization of the pelvic organs and is a less awkward procedure for both the operator and the patient. On the other hand, culdoscopy is a simpler procedure requiring less equipment and usually providing a satisfactory solution to a diagnostic pelvic problem. The principal indications for culdoscopy are unexplained acute or chronic pelvic pain, unexplained infertility, amenorrhea with uncertainty as to the status of the ovaries, and clarification as to the presence or absence of a pelvic mass and its origin. This method is particularly helpful in the differentiation between tubal pregnancy, pelvic inflammatory disease, and a hematoma of the ovary. It has also been useful in differentiating between a serous uterine leiomyoma and an enlarged ovary. However, if a clear-cut adnexal mass is present, exploratory laparotomy would be the preferred approach. The main value of culdoscopy is to reveal negative or insignificant findings, thus avoiding a major operative procedure. Only one of ten culdoscopies at our institution has revealed findings justifying major operative intervention. Sedation with local, spinal, or general anesthesia may be used; an intratracheal tube should be used with general anesthesia.

Technique. With the patient in the lithotomy position, a rectovaginal examination is performed before surgical preparation to make certain that the cul-de-sac is free, that the uterine fundus is mobile, and that no mass is present. Routine surgical preparation and draping are carried out, the bladder is emptied, and a No. 14 Foley catheter is placed in the cervical canal and its bulb distended so that indigo carmine dye may be instilled if desired. The catheter is tucked into the vagina, a sponge is inserted, and the patient is placed in the knee-chest position. We place the thighs parallel to upright stirrups, put a cushioned armboard between the lower thighs and stirrups, and place a wide belt around the thighs, stirrups, and ends of the armboard. The thighs must be perpendicular to the operating table, and the abdomen must be elevated above the table so that its contents are not pressed into the pelvis. Povidone-iodine solution is applied to the genital area again, and drapes are placed.

A Heaney retractor elevates the posterior vaginal wall, and a tenaculum is placed on the posterior cervix close to its vaginal junction (Fig. 17). The cervix is depressed downward, thereby stretching the uterosacral ligamènts and defining the point for a quick thrust of the trocar into the cul-de-sac — a point 2 cm above the midline of the cervicovaginal junction (Fig. 18). As the trocar is removed from its sheath, a rush of air into the abdominal cavity confirms entry into the cul-de-sac. The distal end of the culdoscope is placed in hot water to prevent its lens from becoming fogged within the pelvis. At this point, the retractor may be removed, but the tenaculum is left in place on the cervix. Manipulation of the tenaculum and pressure on the lower abdomen by an assistant may permit improved visualization as necessary. With tubes and ovaries in view, diluted indigo carmine dye may be instilled by a No. 20 needle into the Foley catheter, which has been sealed at its end with a clamp. After the examination is completed, the sheath is left in place until the patient is returned to the prone position, so that excess air is expelled from the abdomen before the sheath is removed.

Postoperative Considerations. The patient's respiratory status is carefully monitored before the endotracheal tube is removed. Intravenous fluids are discontinued after the patient is alert. The patient may be up and take a diet as tolerated (usually liquids) and may be discharged later in the day or the next morning. Only mild pain medication is required.

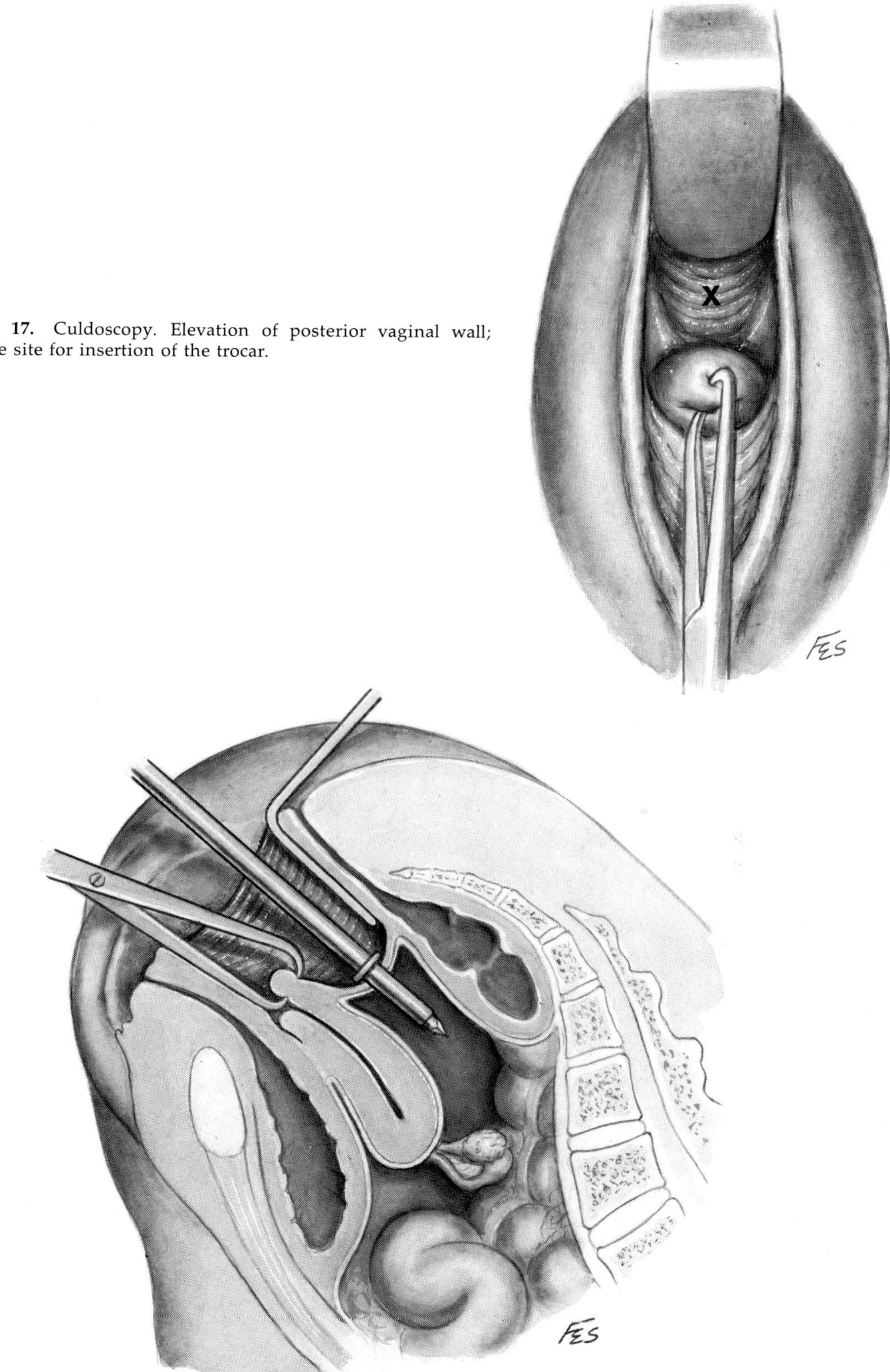

Figure 17. Culdoscopy. Elevation of posterior vaginal wall; **X** marks the site for insertion of the trocar.

Figure 18. Culdoscopy. The posterior vaginal fornix is placed under tension by depressing the cervix. The trocar is inserted with a quick thrust about 2 cm from the posterior cervicovaginal junction.

COLPOTOMY

Comments. The indications for colpotomy are the same as those for culdoscopy and laparoscopy, but it has the advantage of direct palpation and direct visualization of the pelvic organs. Although it does permit direct removal of a tube or ovary, such procedures should be undertaken only by the most experienced vaginal surgeons. In our present practice colpotomy has become a rare procedure, being performed only when the culdoscope and laparoscope are not available.

Technique. Before colpotomy is undertaken, examination must disclose no mass in the cul-de-sac, and the uterus must be mobile. A tenaculum is placed on the posterior cervix near its junction with the vagina. The cervix is pushed up, while countertraction is maintained by a posterior retractor (Fig. 19 *A*). A 1 cm incision is made between the uterosacral ligaments about 2 cm from the cervicovaginal junction. Once in the cul-de-sac, it is preferable to stretch the opening wider manually rather than to use the knife or scissors. If more exposure is necessary, the uterosacral ligaments can be divided and ligated, as would be done for a vaginal hysterectomy. At this point, it is useful to insert a finger to palpate the uterus and adnexa; the diagnosis is often clarified by this simple maneuver. A Heaney retractor is placed in the cul-de-sac beneath the uterus and angled from side to side to permit exposure of the tube and ovary on each side (Fig. 19 *B*). Long instruments are helpful for grasping the tube and ovary, but it is important to avoid tearing the tissues, since quick access to their blood supply is limited through this approach. If partial removal of a tube or ovary is contemplated, it is brought down to the operative opening with a long ovum clamp (Babcock intestinal clamp, 9.5 inch or 24.13 cm), and a suture (Ethicon C123 chromic catgut 2–0) is placed in the ovary for exposure and later used as the beginning of a continuous locking suture. Long Allis clamps are placed on the tissue to be removed (Fig. 20 *A*), and a wedge of tissue is removed (Fig. 20 *B*), placing a continuous locking suture after each 0.5 to 1 cm division of tissue (Fig. 20 *C*). The technique used for tubal sterilization should be flexible according to the degree of surgical exposure. If the isthmus of the tube can be mobilized, a simple ligature of the tube is performed with 2–0 chromic catgut with removal of the loop of tube beyond the ligature. If only the distal portion of the tube may be mobilized with ease, it may be ligated as far as possible medially with chromic catgut and removed. The colpotomy site is closed with simple chromic catgut (Ethicon U246 chromic catgut 1–0) through mucosa and peritoneum, closing the lateral angles first (Fig. 20 *D* and *E*).

Postoperative Considerations. The vaginal pack is removed two hours after operation. The bladder is catheterized only as necessary. Intravenous fluids are discontinued after the patient is awake and alert and has normal vital signs. Hemoglobin and hematocrit determinations are checked the day after operation. The patient may be up and have a regular diet as tolerated. Codeine, 60 mg orally or subcutaneously, is given every four hours as necessary for pain. The patient can be discharged on the first or second postoperative day and should be told to avoid tampons, douches, and coitus. The patient should also avoid strenuous activity for two weeks after a diagnostic colpotomy and for four weeks if operative excision of the tube or ovary or both was performed.

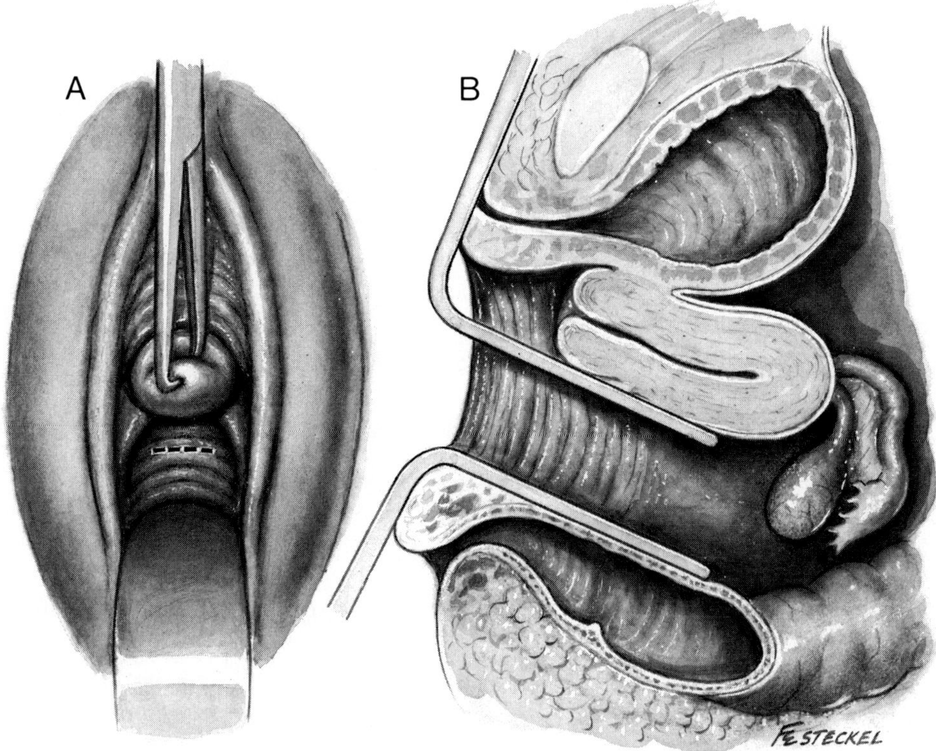

Figure 19. Colpotomy. *A,* Posterior fornix of vagina is exposed and placed under tension before making a 1 cm transverse incision (dashed line) about 2 cm from the cervicovaginal junction. *B,* Heaney retractors are used to provide exposure.

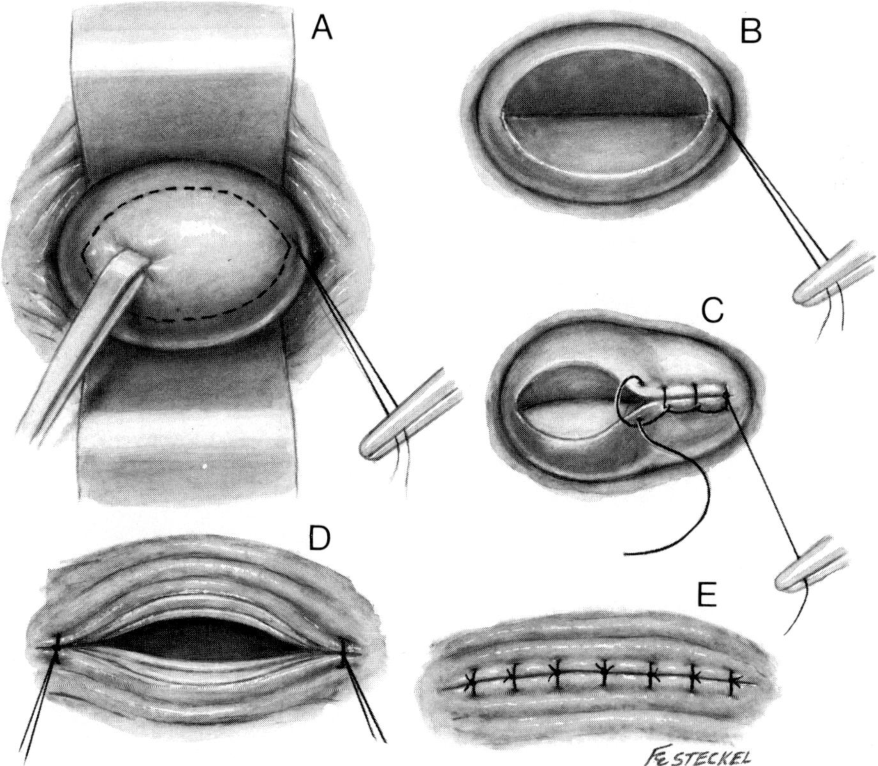

Figure 20. A tension suture is placed at one end of the ovary before wedge biopsy and closure of defect with a locking suture (*A* through *C*). Starting with the angles, the incision is closed with sutures through the mucosa and peritoneum (*D* and *E*).

COLPOTOMY FOR DRAINAGE OF AN ABSCESS

Comments. Drainage of a large midline pelvic abscess dissecting the rectovaginal septum is a rare but useful application of colpotomy.

Technique. A simple incision is made in the upper posterior vaginal midline in the center of the fluctuant abscess. The opening is stretched larger with a clamp, and a finger or instrument is *gently* employed to explore the abscess cavity, breaking up any adhesions or sacculation. A sample is taken for culture of aerobic and anaerobic organisms. A No. 18 mushroom catheter is inserted into the abscess cavity and anchored with a 1–0 chromic catgut suture if necessary.

Postoperative Considerations. The head of the bed is elevated 30 degrees. The catheter is connected to low suction drainage and 1 per cent neomycin sulfate solution, 20 cc, is instilled every eight hours, and the catheter is clamped for one hour after each instillation. The amount of neomycin is reduced to 10 cc on the second postoperative day, to 5 cc on the third postoperative day, and it is discontinued on the fourth postoperative day. On the sixth postoperative day or after the patient has been afebrile for 48 hours, the catheter is removed. The parenteral and oral use of antibiotics and the dosages must be individualized. Some patients improve dramatically after the colpotomy, indicating that the single abscess was the main problem. In other patients it may only be a part of a generalized pelvic infection, and intensive antibiotic therapy must be continued and guided by culture results. A suprapubic catheter is maintained in the bladder until the vaginal catheter has been removed and ambulation is permitted.

Major Vulvovaginal Surgery

VAGINAL REPAIR

Comments.   Surgical treatment for prolapse and vaginal relaxation has been, in my opinion, the biggest source of unnecessary gynecologic surgery. The medical profession has cultivated a myth regarding the need to repair the natural loss of vaginal support that results from childbearing, aging, and congenital or acquired weakness of the pelvic supports. Repeated inquiry among a multitude of patients suggests that the operation is often performed because the physician said it was necessary. Too many repairs and vaginal hysterectomies have been performed when simple reassurance or physiotherapy would have sufficed. When the patient has urinary problems or pressure symptoms, it is important to establish a connection to the finding of pelvic relaxation and to judge the overall significance of the symptoms for the patient's health. If the symptoms are severe enough to curtail the patient's daily activities, then operation should be considered providing no medical contraindications are present and childbearing is complete. When operation is performed, the tendency is to do too extensive a repair, with resulting compromise of vaginal function. It is far better to convert a third-degree rectocele into a first-degree one than to create perfect support now and a dyspareunia problem 10 years later. Conversely, in the very elderly patient with no desire for vaginal function, it is wise to do the most expedient repair to accomplish the best result in the shortest operative time, even though vaginal closure results. Vaginal relaxation and prolapse are manifested in many different forms, so that the basic techniques must often be modified to serve the needs of the individual patient.

Special instruments for vaginal surgery include two Heaney needle holders; two Heaney clamps; short, medium, and deep weighted vaginal retractors; and a long Babcock intestinal 9.5 inch (24.13 cm) clamp. A ⅝ circle needle (Davis & Geck TT3 Dexon 1–0 or Ethicon U246 chromic catgut 1–0) is very helpful for the suspension stitches and for closure of the peritoneum and the vagina. A suction tube is employed during all operations.

Technique.   The genital area and lower abdomen are prepared and draped. The bladder is emptied with a straight catheter. To reduce blood loss, a 1 to 200,000 solution of epinephrine may be injected beneath the mucosa in the midline from the introitus to the apex of the vagina. If the cervix is absent, a small vertical mucosal incision is begun with the scalpel at the level of the vesicourethral junction; the mucosa is undermined superficially in the midline proximally to the vaginal apex and distally beneath the urethra (Figs. 21 and 22). Allis clamps or straight Ochsner clamps are used to place the mucosa under tension. If the cervix is present, a short transverse mucosal incision is made at the anterior cervicovaginal junction, and this is used as a starting point for undermining the mucosa distally to the urethra. The same basic technique applies to the posterior repair for a relaxed vaginal outlet, rectocele, and enterocele, except that a small triangle of mucosa is excised at the posterior aspect of the introitus in the case of the posterior vaginal repair.

Our technique as reported in the chapter in *Lewis-Walters Practice of Surgery* has been revised. It is preferable to begin all such repairs by placing small pursestring sutures (Ethicon G123 chromic catgut 2–0 or Davis & Geck T5 Dexon 3–0) at the top or dome of the cystocele (Figs. 23 and 24), enterocele (Figs. 25 and 26), or rectocele (Fig. 27). Although this area of the relaxed bladder, rectum, or cul-de-sac is thin and weak, the pursestring suture can be used to strengthen the repair further and to close dead space. A cystocele may require one pursestring suture; a rectocele, two; and an enterocele, four. After appropriate inversion of the tissue with the pursestring sutures, standard plicating sutures (Ethicon U246 chromic catgut 1–0) are used to bring together the stronger lateral tissue to complete the repair. Caution should be exercised to avoid "overrepair" of a cystocele, for incontinence can result. Plicating sutures should be placed beneath the urethra, and a gap should be left between the repair of the urethrocele and the repair of the cystocele (Fig. 24). A reinforcing second plicating suture may be appropriate for the vesicourethral angle, or the standard double plication or pubococcygeoplasty **may** be used when urinary stress incontinence is present (see section on correction of urinary stress incontinence). Redundant mucosa is trimmed, and the anterior mucosa is approximated with simple or vertical mattress sutures.

In the presence of a relaxed vaginal outlet associated with an enterocele and a rectocele, a small triangle of mucosa is excised at the posterior introitus, and the mucosa is undermined in the posterior midline to the apex of the vault or to the cervicovaginal junction if the cervix is present. A pursestring suture with 2–0 chromic catgut is placed superfically around the tip of the enterocele (Fig. 25); the tip is inverted with a Kelly clamp or with a finger as the suture is tied. Pursestring sutures are used to invert the enterocele (Fig. 26) and the rectocele (Fig. 27). Simple plicating sutures of 1–0 chromic catgut are used to cover the inverted enterocele and rectocele with stronger tissue (Fig. 28). At the posterior outlet the levator fascia is plicated with a single or double layer of sutures according to the degree of relaxation present. Although some gynecologic surgeons prefer to incise the fascia and approximate the levator muscle separately with such a plication, it is not believed necessary to do so. The final closure of the perineum is made with a simple or continuous subcuticular 1–0 chromic catgut or polyglycolic acid suture (Fig. 29).

Whenever an indwelling bladder catheter is required for longer than 24 hours, a Dow Corning suprapubic Silastic No. 12 Cystocath is employed. The bladder is again emptied with a straight catheter, and sterile saline solution, 400 to 500 cc, is instilled. The round shield is cemented to the skin with its center at a point 3 cm above the symphysis pubis, where the needle with a trocar is inserted first to the rectus fascia and then with a firm thrust into the bladder; successful implantation is confirmed by the free flow of saline through the hollowed portion of the trocar. The trocar is removed, the Silastic catheter is inserted for two thirds of its length into the bladder, and the metal sheath is removed. The catheter is attached to the central device and anchored to the plastic shield. It is important to tape the catheter from the shield to the drainage attachment to avoid kinking and cutting of the Silastic tubing; it is also advisable to tape or suture the shield securely to the skin.

Postoperative Considerations. A vaginal pack (1 inch gauze) is removed routinely in two hours but is kept in overnight if oozing has been excessive. Prophylactic antibiotics are employed routinely. If a suprapubic catheter has been used, the patient is allowed to void on the fourth postoperative day with the catheter open, provided that she has been afebrile for 24 hours. With the suprapubic catheter we find a low residual urine, which the patient may void. On the fifth postoperative day the catheter is turned off during the daytime and opened for discomfort or for measurement of residual urine at six-hour intervals. One must be alert to the occasional blockage of the delicate Silastic catheter as a result of tearing, twisting, or kinking and to its obstruction by bladder sediment and mucosa; inspection, irrigation, and advancement of the catheter usually solve the problem. Rarely the catheter may pass through the urethra with the urine; in such patients the catheter is cut with a sterile scissors flush with the urethral orifice and withdrawn from above back into the bladder. Prolonged urinary retention is not seen with a routine repair but may occur with extensive operations for incontinence, as will be discussed later in the text.

The patient usually progresses to a normal diet on the day after operation and is allowed to ambulate as desired. The patient may be discharged six to seven days after operation.

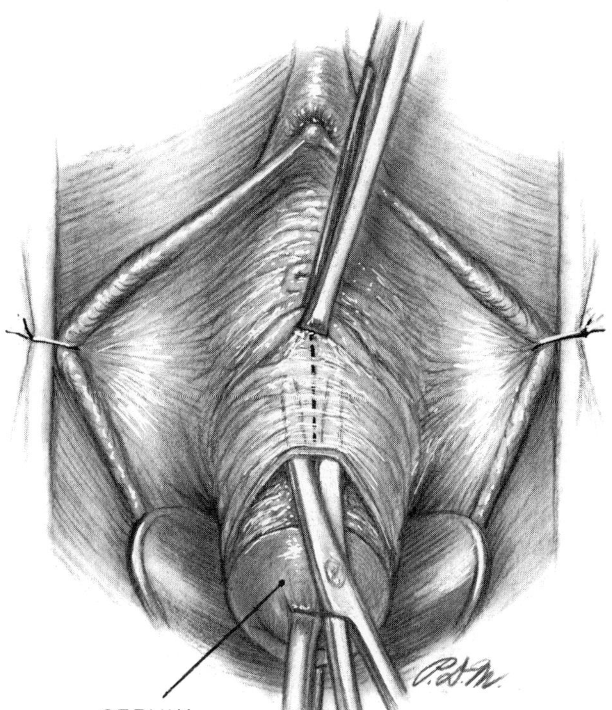

Figure 21. Cystocele repair. Undermining the mucosa.

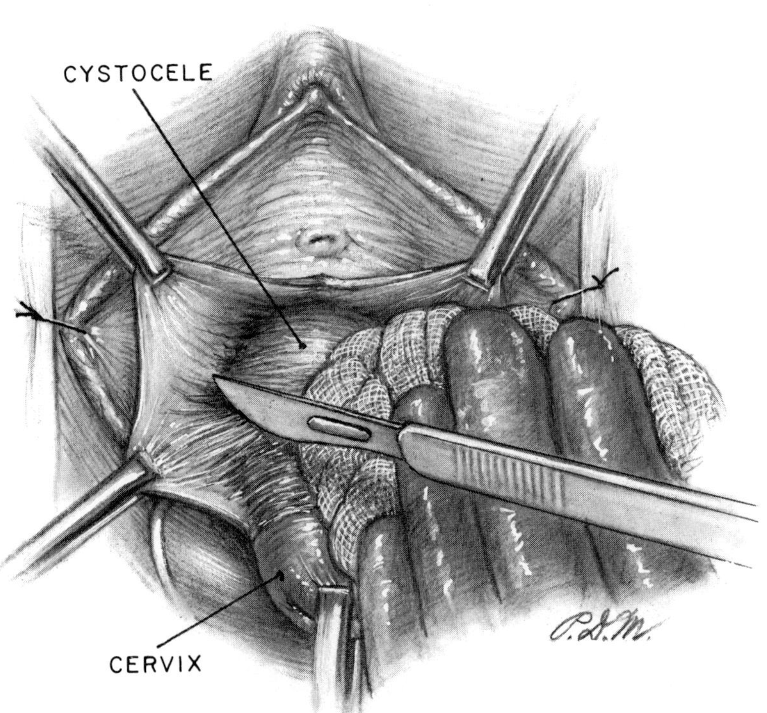

Figure 22. Cystocele repair. Further separation of the mucosa from the cystocele.

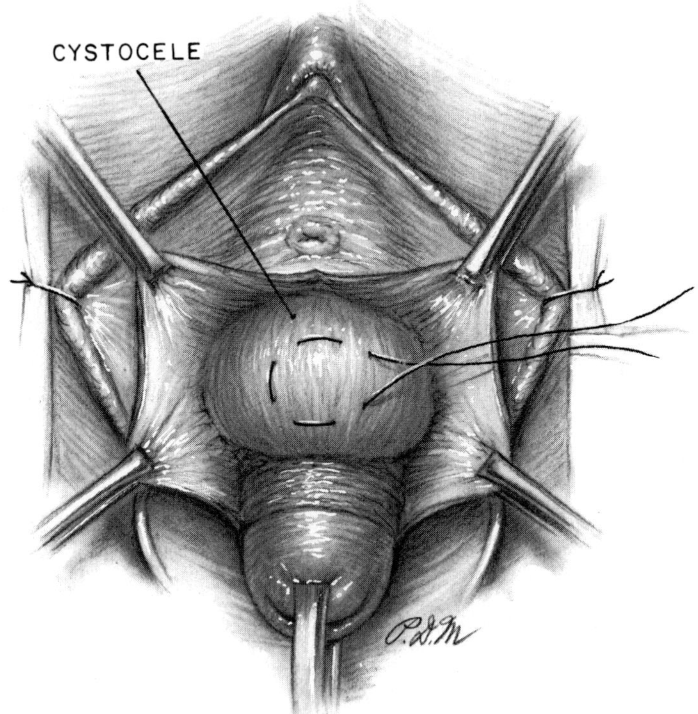

Figure 23. Cystocele repair. Superficial placement of pursestring suture around dome of the cystocele.

Figure 24. Cystocele repair. Plication of vesicourethral angle leaving a small gap between it and plication of the cystocele.

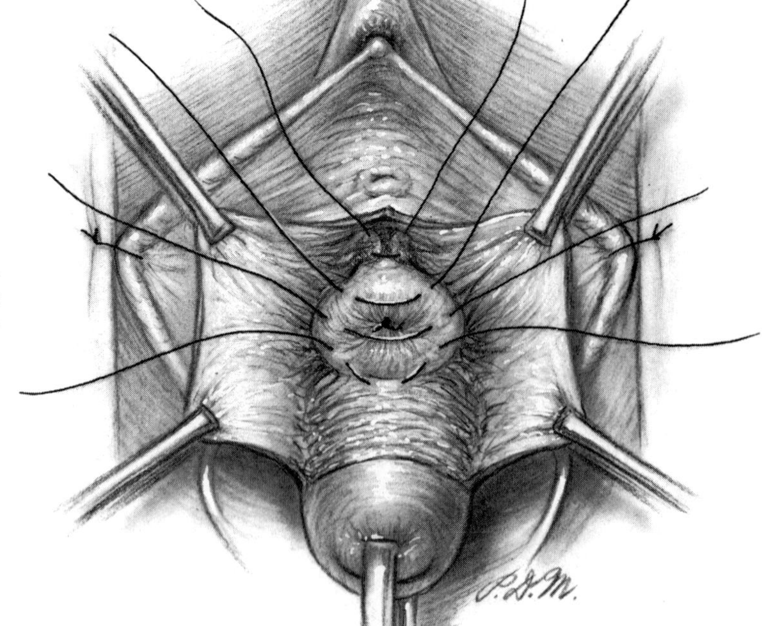

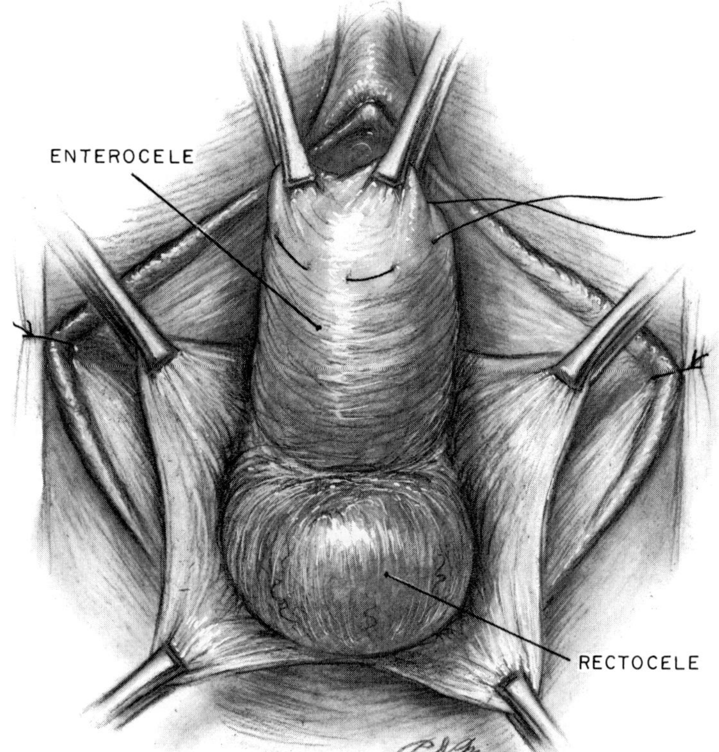

Figure 25. Enterocele-rectocele repair. The mucosa has been undermined from the introitus to the top of the vagina, and a superficial pursestring suture has been placed around the tip of the enterocele.

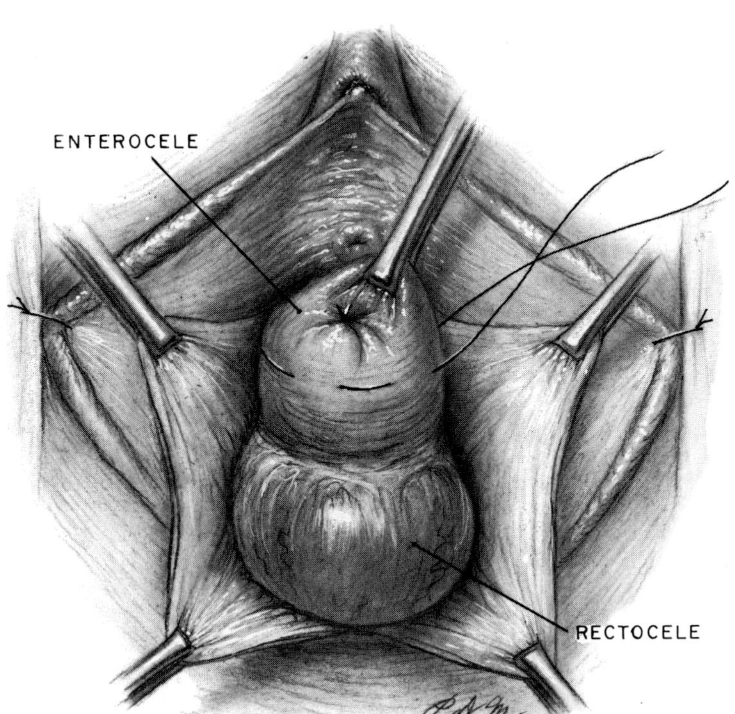

Figure 26. Enterocele-rectocele repair. Inversion of the enterocele with a series of pursestring sutures.

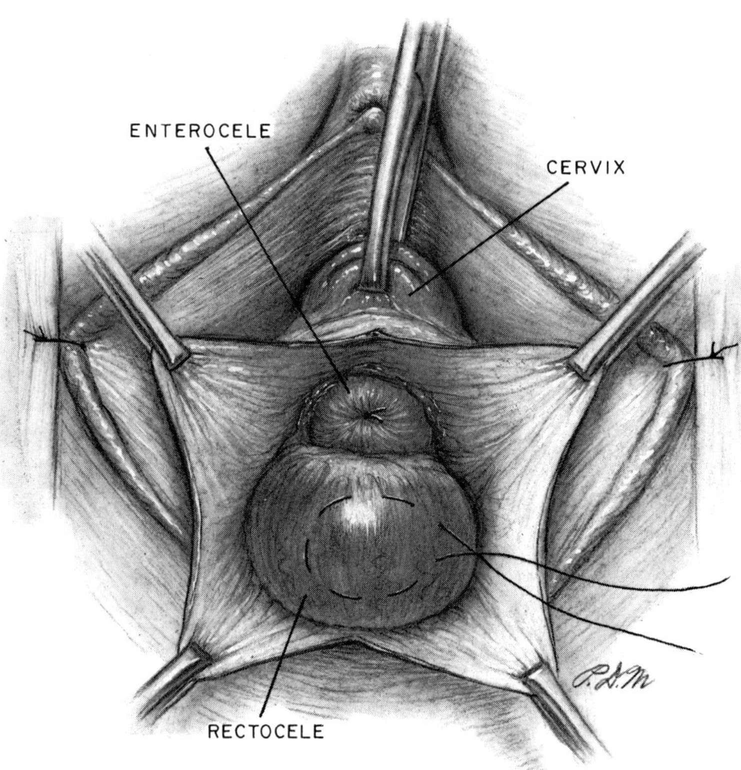

Figure 27. Enterocele-rectocele repair. Similar superficial pursestring sutures are employed to initiate rectocele repair.

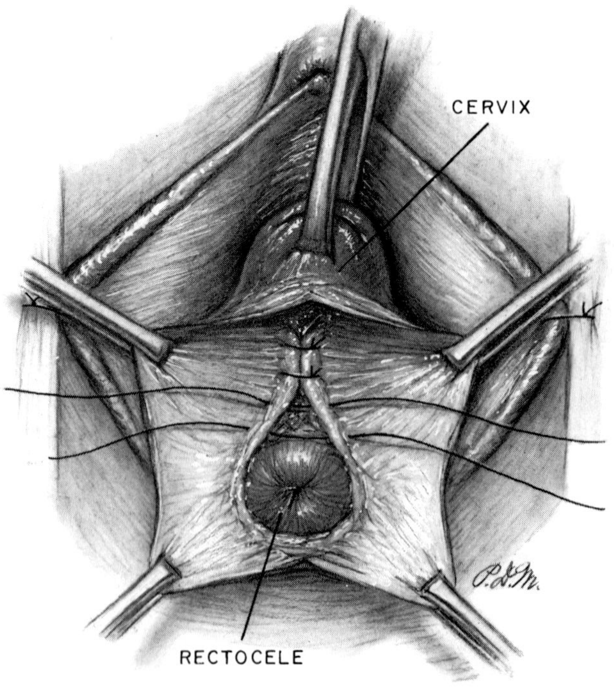

Figure 28. Enterocele-rectocele repair. Simple plicating sutures are used to bring the stronger tissue over the inverted enterocele and rectocele.

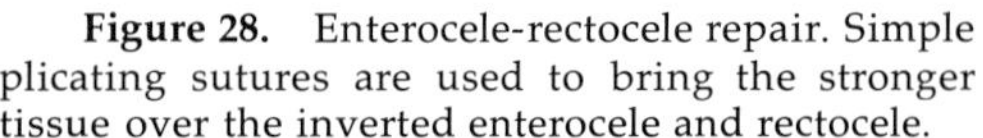

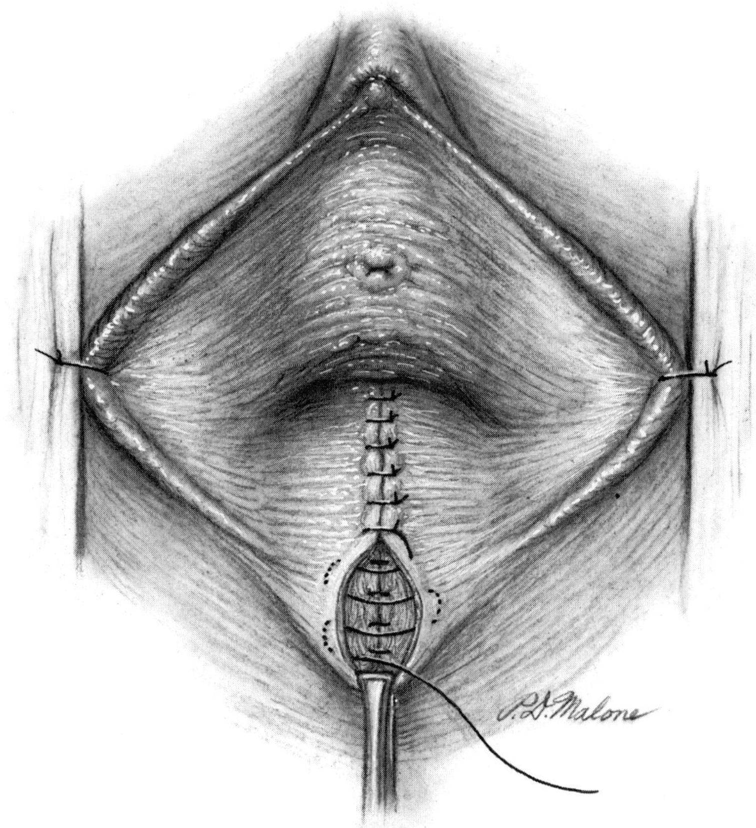

Figure 29. Repair of relaxed vaginal outlet. The levator muscle and fascia have been plicated with simple sutures in a single or double layer, and the mucosa with adjacent perineal skin is approximated with a continuous submucosal or subcuticular suture.

COLPOCLEISIS

Partial Colpocleisis with the Uterus Present (Le Fort Procedure)

Comments. Partial colpocleisis should be reserved for the elderly patient who has no prospect of coitus. It offers the best result with reduced operating time and fewer complications. On the other hand, the ability to detect future disease of the uterus is compromised. Naturally, in such patients use of a pessary (the Gellhorn is preferred) deserves consideration before surgical treatment is contemplated.

Technique. Equal rectangular sections of vaginal mucosa are excised from the anterior and posterior vagina beginning 2 cm away from the cervical os and making certain that the excision does not extend closer than 4 cm to the external urethral orifice (Fig. 30). The rectangular sections are approximated with simple sutures (Fig. 31). Before the final central mucosal sutures are placed, a limited anterior and posterior repair is carried out between the site of colpocleisis and the introitus (Fig. 32), thus correcting the distal component of the prolapse. The instruments and sutures used are the same as those for vaginal repair.

Postoperative Considerations. Intravenous fluids are continued until the morning after operation, at which time the No. 14 5 cc Foley catheter is removed and the patient may be out of bed and have a normal diet. Discharge is usually planned for the third postoperative day.

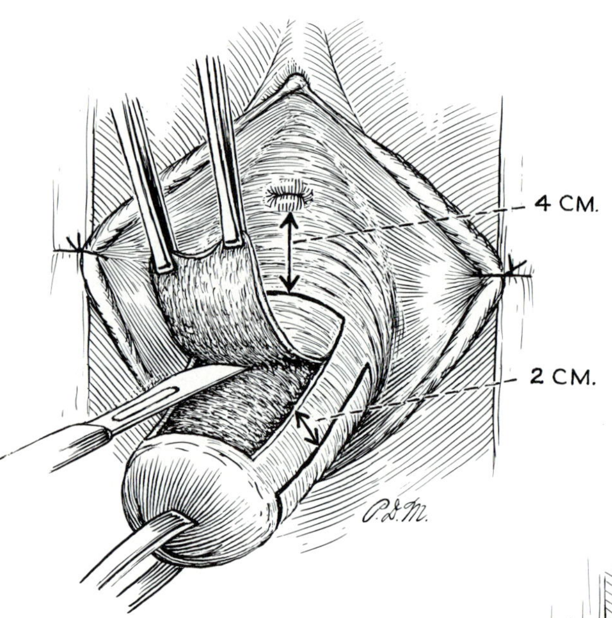

Figure 30. Partial colpocleisis (Le Fort procedure). Excision of rectangular sections of vaginal mucosa. (From Copenhaver, EH: Abnormalities of pelvic support. *In* Lewis-Walters Practice of Surgery, Vol 10, Chapter 21. Hagerstown, Md, W F Prior Co, Inc, 1966, p 22.)

Figure 31. Partial colpocleisis (Le Fort procedure). Approximation of denuded areas with simple sutures. (From Copenhaver, EH: Abnormalities of pelvic support. *In* Lewis-Walters Practice of Surgery, Vol 10, Chapter 21. Hagerstown, Md, W F Prior Co, Inc, 1966, p 22.)

Figure 32. Partial colpocleisis (Le Fort procedure). A limited repair is performed for the distal 4 cm of anterior and posterior relaxation before final closure of the mucosa; lateral tunnels remain extending to the cervix. (From Copenhaver, EH: Abnormalities of pelvic support. *In* Lewis-Walters Practice of Surgery, Vol 10, Chapter 21. Hagerstown, Md, W F Prior Co, Inc, 1966, p 22.)

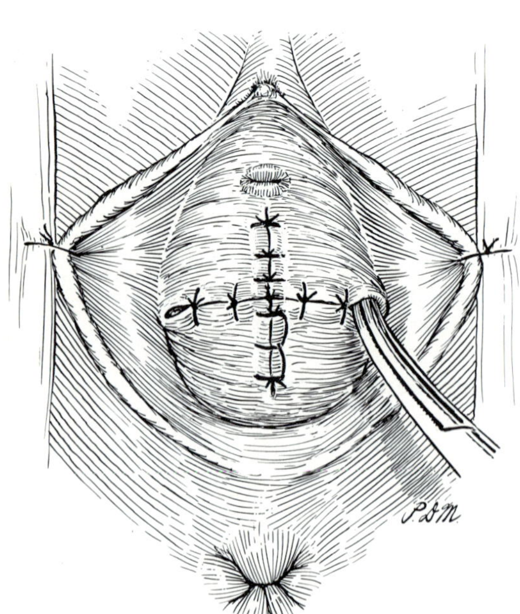

Subtotal Colpocleisis for Vaginal Prolapse

Comments. Subtotal colpocleisis, like the Le Fort procedure, assumes that the patient has no prospect of coitus. In such patients it is the procedure of choice for management of severe prolapse of the vaginal vault, for it achieves the best result with a short operating time.

Technique. The prolapsed vaginal apex is held with Allis clamps while the mucosa is excised in quadrants extending to within 4 cm of the urethral orifice and the introitus (Fig. 33). The small fragment of mucosa held by the clamps is excised before pursestring closure of the vagina is begun. Pursestring sutures close the vagina (Fig. 34), the peritoneal cavity is not opened, and a limited anterior and posterior repair is performed to correct the lower 4 cm of prolapsed vagina. The instruments and sutures used are the same as those for vaginal repair.

Postoperative Considerations. The postoperative care is the same as that for patients who have undergone the Le Fort procedure. However, since this operation is more extensive, a suprapubic catheter may be used and the patient tapered off the catheter on the third or fourth postoperative day before discharge from the hospital on the fifth or sixth day after operation.

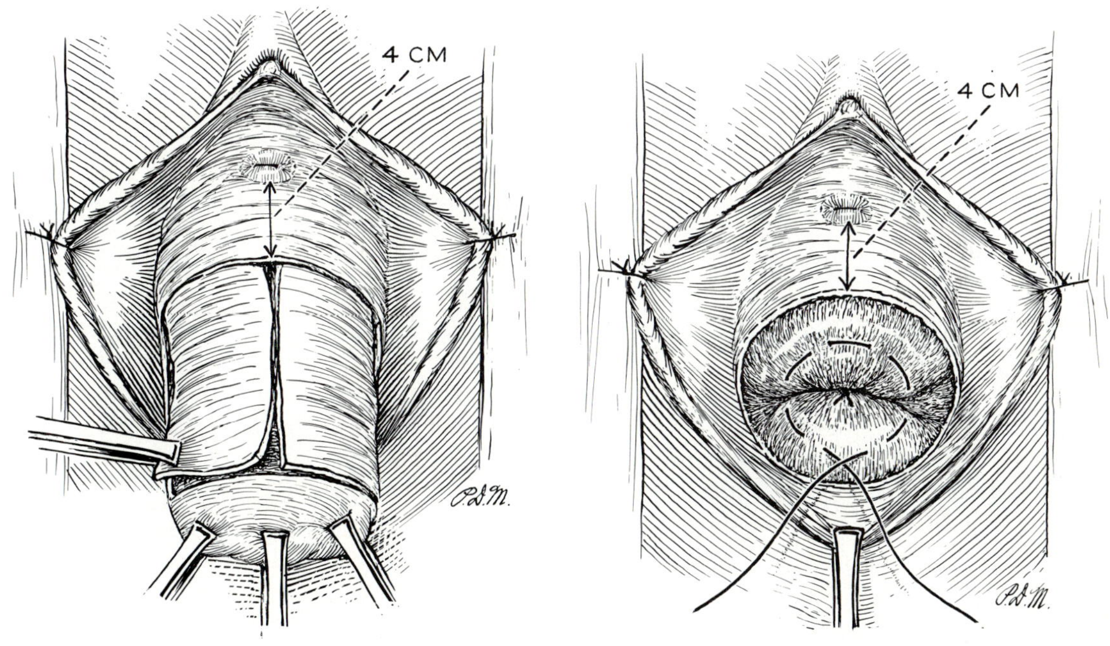

Figure 33.   **Figure 34.**

Figure 33. Subtotal colpocleisis. Superficial excision of vaginal mucosa. (From Copenhaver, EH: Abnormalities of pelvic support. *In* Lewis-Walters Practice of Surgery, Vol 10, Chapter 21, Hagerstown, Md, W F Prior Co, Inc, 1966, p 23.)

Figure 34. Subtotal colpocleisis. Inversion of prolapsed vagina with pursestring sutures. (From Copenhaver, EH: Abnormalities of pelvic support. *In* Lewis-Walters Practice of Surgery, Vol 10, Chapter 21. Hagerstown, Md, W F Prior Co, Inc, 1966, p 24.)

Apical Colpocleisis with Repair for Vaginal Prolapse

Comments. In contrast to the preceding procedures for colpocleisis, apical colpocleisis with repair is formidable and time consuming. The objective is to preserve vaginal function while taking only a vaginal approach to the correction of severe prolapse of the vagina coexistent with a hysterectomy for uterine prolapse or after a much earlier hysterectomy. Such an operation involves creative reconstruction of the vagina and differs for every patient. It brings into play all the facets of vaginal repair, together with a minimal sacrifice of vaginal mucosa. This procedure *does* reduce the caliber and length of the vagina, even in the best of hands. If more depth and caliber are desirable, an abdominal suspension of the vagina should be combined with abdominal closure of the cul-de-sac or a limited vaginal repair or both. Like radical pelvic surgery, this procedure requires the most experienced and skillful of gynecologic surgeons.

Technique. When the procedure is contemplated as an immediate sequel to vaginal hysterectomy or vaginal removal of a cervical stump, a 2 cm ring of mucosa is excised adjacent to the cervix (Fig. 35, *inset*) at the beginning of the operation in preparation for a partial colpocleisis. An extensive vaginal repair is performed with removal of only narrow strips of redundant mucosa (Fig. 35).

When vaginal vault prolapse is treated in the absence of the uterus, the vaginal mucosa is undermined and separated from the underlying cystocele, rectocele, or enterocele (Fig. 36) in a manner similar to that for subtotal colpocleisis described in the preceding section, except that the mucosa is not excised. Instead, several pursestring sutures are employed to invert the apex of the prolapsed submucosal tissue (Fig. 37), and any strong adjacent tissue or ligaments are attached to this inverted portion of the repair. A limited anterior and posterior repair is performed, maintaining the mucosa intact or making a simple vertical midline incision of the mucosa for exposure. Narrow hourglass-shaped strips of mucosa are removed. At this point the anterior and posterior apex of the vaginal mucosa is resuspended to the partial colpocleisis produced by the previously placed pursestring sutures (Fig. 38). This serves to recreate a vagina of shorter but adequate length. The mucosa is approximated transversely at the apex and vertically in the anterior and posterior midlines with interrupted sutures down to the perineum, where a routine perineorrhaphy is performed (Fig. 39 and see section on vaginal repair). The end result is the same as in apical colpocleisis with vaginal hysterectomy and repair. A severe prolapse of the vagina is transformed into a shortened and narrowed vagina with first-degree relaxation — not a perfect result but a functional one. The instruments and sutures used here are the same as those employed for vaginal repair.

Postoperative Considerations. Postoperative considerations are the same as those described in the section on vaginal repair. A vaginal pack is inserted and retained until the morning after operation. A suprapubic catheter is used. Prophylactic antibiotics are usually given because of the extensive nature of the repair.

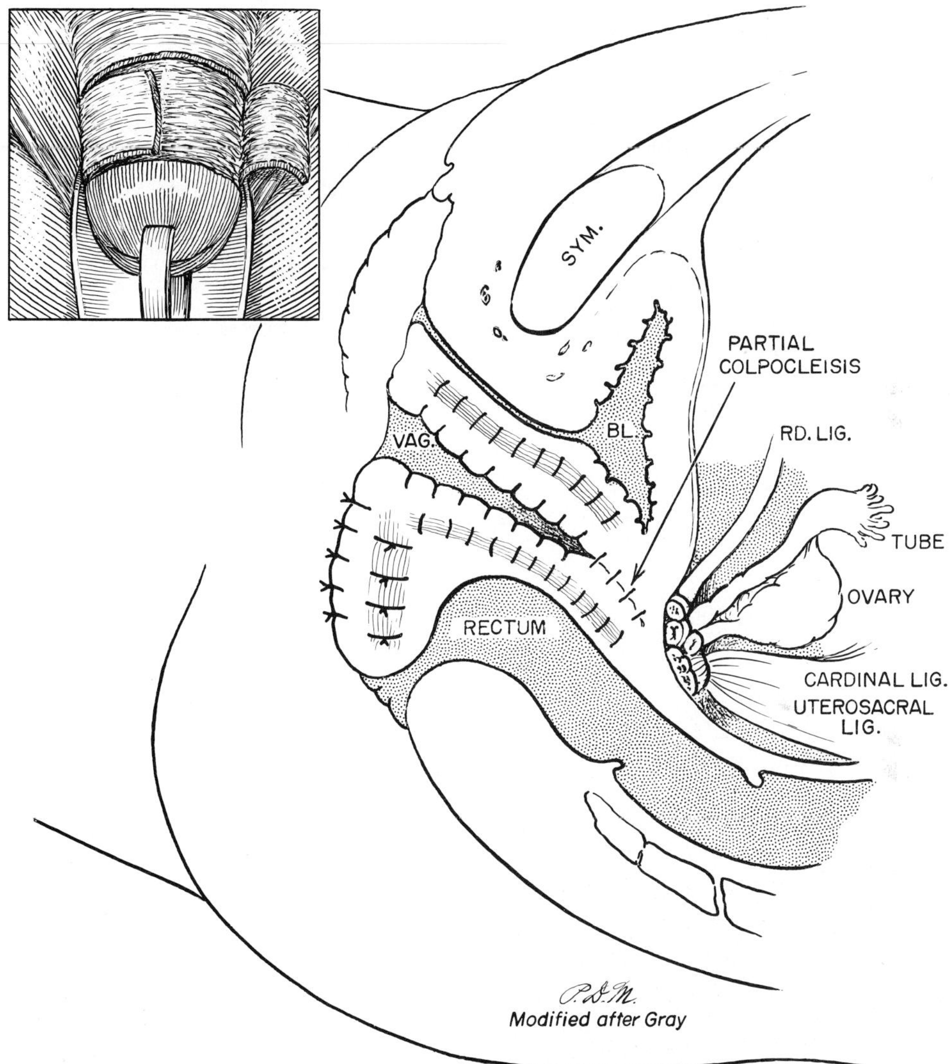

Figure 35. Apical colpocleisis with vaginal hysterectomy and repair. Initial removal of 2 cm rim of mucosa (*inset*) before routine vaginal hysterectomy and limited repair, with end result depicted. (From Copenhaver, EH: Abnormalities of pelvic support. *In* Lewis-Walters Practice of Surgery, Vol. 10, Chapter 21. Hagerstown, Md, W F Prior Co, Inc, 1966, p 20.)

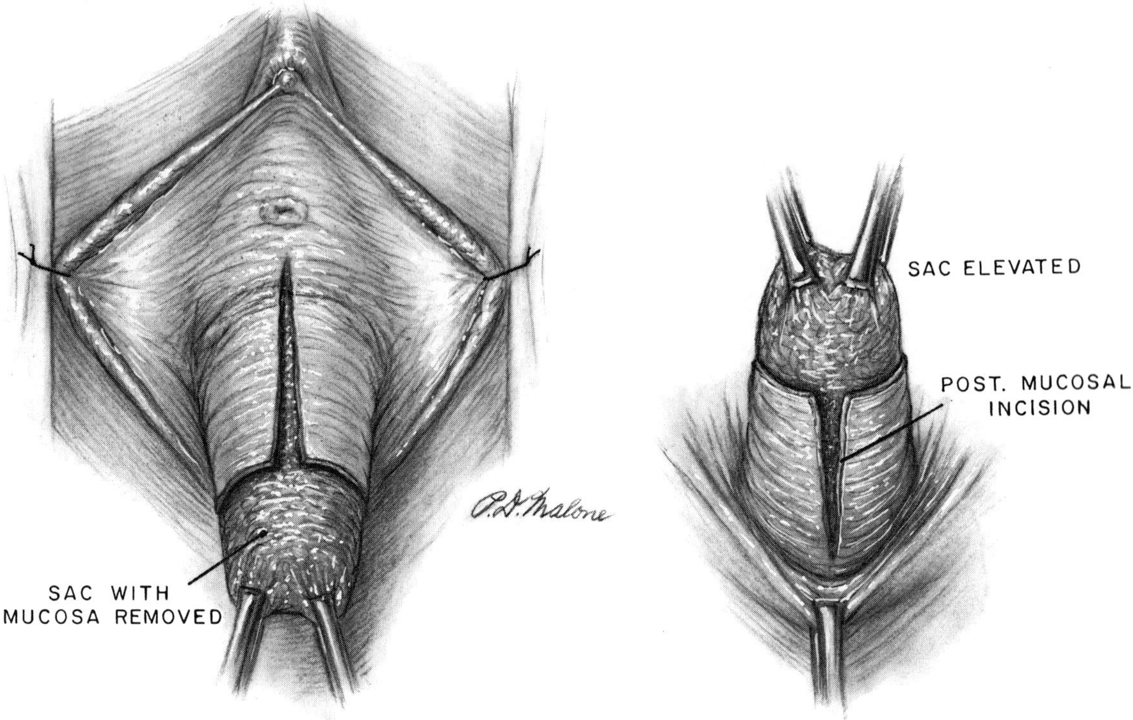

Figure 36.   Apical colpocleisis with repair. Apical mucosa has been excised and repair initiated.

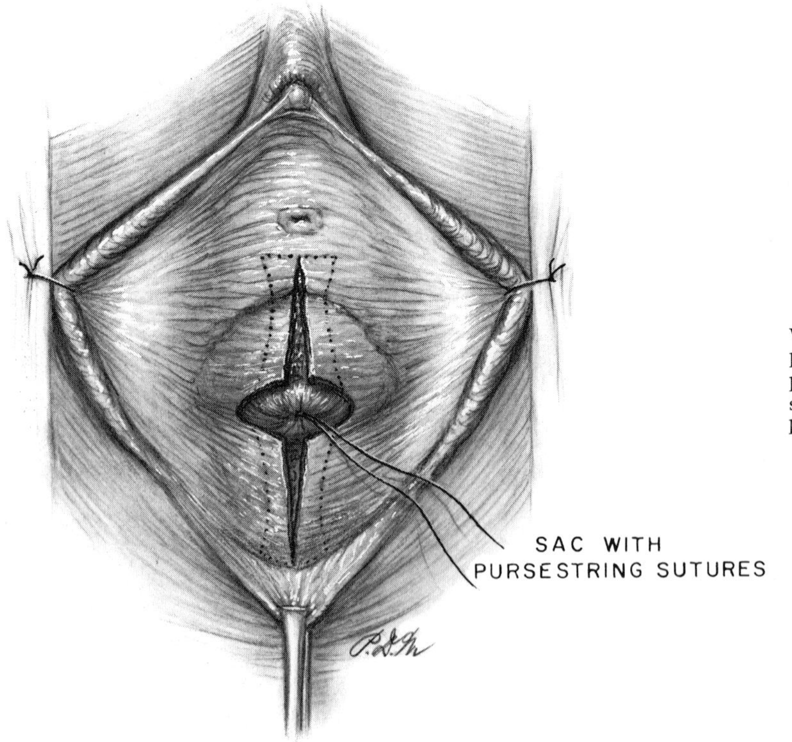

Figure 37.   Apical colpocleisis with repair. The distal portion of the prolapse has been inverted with pursestring sutures, and narrow strips of vaginal mucosa are outlined for excision.

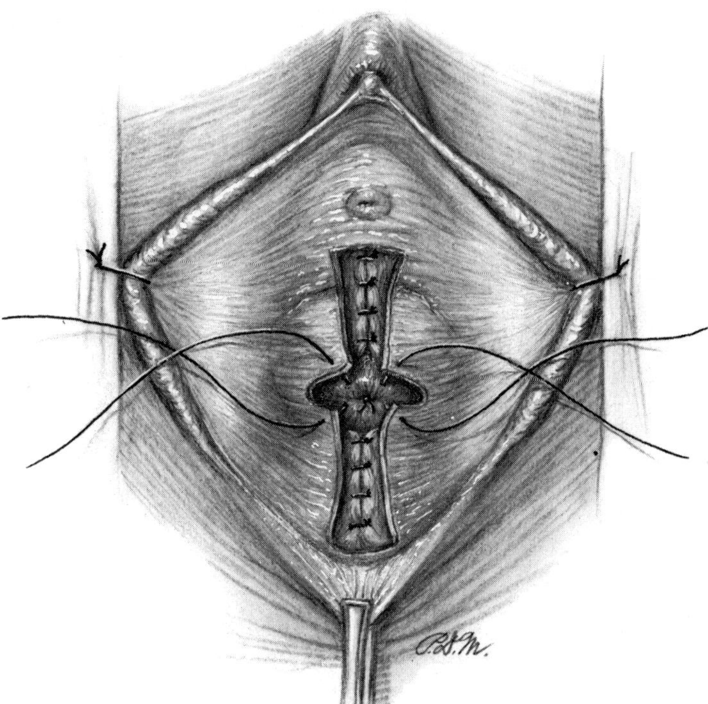

Figure 38. Apical colpocleisis with repair. After a routine anterior and posterior plication, the apical edges of the mucosa are suspended to the previously inverted and repaired apex of the vagina.

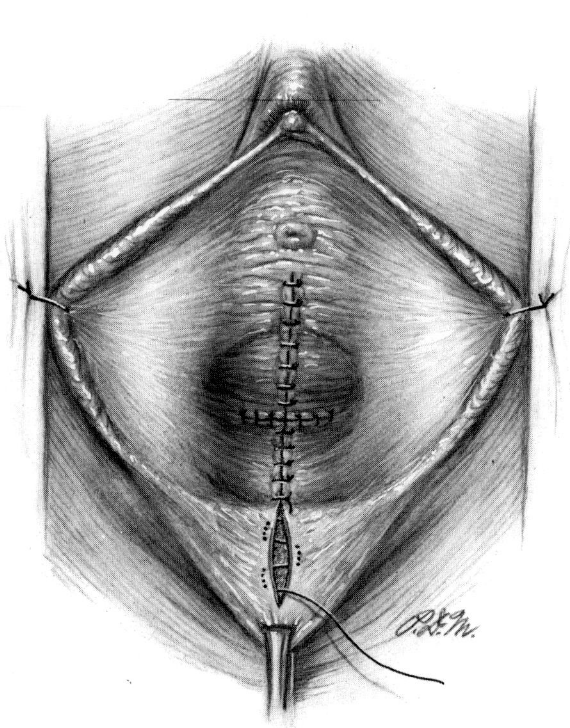

Figure 39. Apical colpocleisis with repair. The mucosa is approximated, and a routine repair of the relaxed vaginal outlet is performed.

CORRECTION OF URINARY STRESS INCONTINENCE

Comments. The purpose of this section is to focus on techniques for the correction of stress incontinence. However, it must be emphasized that a surgical procedure can only correct a mechanical deficiency in urinary control. Therefore, correct diagnosis is important. A cystometric study or a serial radiographic study is not a substitute for careful questioning of the patient. If the incontinence is not precisely the result of stress, if the patient has any history of urinary tract infections, if she experiences any urgency or dribbling, or if a previous operative attempt has been unsuccessful, a complete urologic evaluation should be performed. If it is concluded that the incontinence is "mainly" of the stress type, the patient should be cautioned as to the prospects of benefit from the operation. While caution is in order, the severity of the problem still may justify an attempted operative solution, for many instances of so-called unstable bladder or dyssynergic detrusor dysfunction may be improved by operation.

Numerous reports in the literature outline results of treatment for stress incontinence of urine, yet few classify the degree of incontinence treated. It is my belief that the majority of operations for incontinence are unnecessary from the outset and that mild to moderate degrees of incontinence are often unnecessarily treated surgically, and these operations are often extended to include unnecessary vaginal hysterectomy and repair. Comparative assessment of different procedures is worthless unless a standard degree of stress incontinence is compared. An incidental finding or history of stress incontinence of urine on coughing should not be an indication for operation. For operation to be indicated, such a symptom should be a primary complaint, should limit the patient's daily activities, and should be severe enough to require protection through the wearing of sanitary pads or the addition of absorbent clothing.

Certainly, obesity and respiratory problems should be resolved before an operation for stress incontinence of urine is attempted. Also, if any question remains as to the significance of the symptom, a three-month trial period of exercises consisting of tightening the pubococcygeal muscles that hold back the urine for two minutes twice a day should be encouraged. It is often gratifying to find that the symptom is improved by such conservative measures or that the passage of time has led the patient herself to reconsider the need for major surgery.

When surgery is indicated, what operation should be performed? Green's studies (1975) have indicated that the traditional vaginal approach is useful for simple, straight descent of the urethra with straining in patients with urinary stress incontinence, whereas a vesicourethral suspension, such as the procedure of Marshall, Marchetti, and Krantz, is best for those patients who have a considerable rotation of the urethra, which points upward when the patient is in the supine position. Green's conclusions certainly reflect logic, for anyone who has performed combined vaginal and suprapubic procedures must admit that the retropubic suspension creates a much more decisive vesicourethral angle than does the usual vaginal plication. Indeed, it may be observed routinely that after vaginal repair and plication of the vesicourethral angle, an added retropubic suspension is not only possible but technically may be performed with ease. It may be concluded that if only one operation were available for treating stress incontinence of urine, the retropubic vesicourethral suspension would be best. However, a vaginal approach is favored by many gynecologic surgeons because it is a less traumatic procedure for the patient. The vaginal procedure causes much less discomfort than the abdominal one. For this reason, it is believed better to continue using the vaginal approach as the primary one for treatment of the patient with marked stress incontinence of urine, but at the same time to add a sling of pubococcygeal muscle and fascia, as in the technique of Ingelman-Sundberg, to ensure a proper vesicourethral angle.

When typical stress incontinence of urine recurs or when an abdominal incision must be made for other reasons, the retropubic vesicourethral suspension should be favored. The sling procedure using fascia lata should be employed when other methods have failed or when a retropubic suspension is not feasible.

Double Plication of Vesicourethral Angle

Technique. The vaginal mucosa is undermined beneath the bladder and urethra after a vertical midline incision, such as that used for vaginal repair, is made (Fig. 40 *A*). The undermining should be wide and should permit visualization of the vesicourethral angle for one half of its circumference. To provide better support, the first row of plicating sutures (Ethicon U246 chromic catgut 1–0; Fig. 40 *B*) is tied with four knots at both ends of each plication (modified after the technique of Tauber) to prevent slipping or "pursestringing" of the suture (Fig. 40, *inset*). A second layer of routine 1–0 chromic catgut plicating sutures is placed after the urethra and bladder neck are mobilized further at their junction with the vaginal mucosa (Fig. 40 *C*). Too extensive a repair of an associated cystocele should be avoided, and a gap should be left between the plicating sutures and the cystocele repair. It would be prudent to leave a residual first-degree cystocele. The excess mucosa is excised and the mucosa approximated with polyglycolic acid sutures (Davis & Geck TT3 Dexon 1–0); it is preferable to use vertical mattress sutures in the region of the vesicourethral angle (Fig. 41).

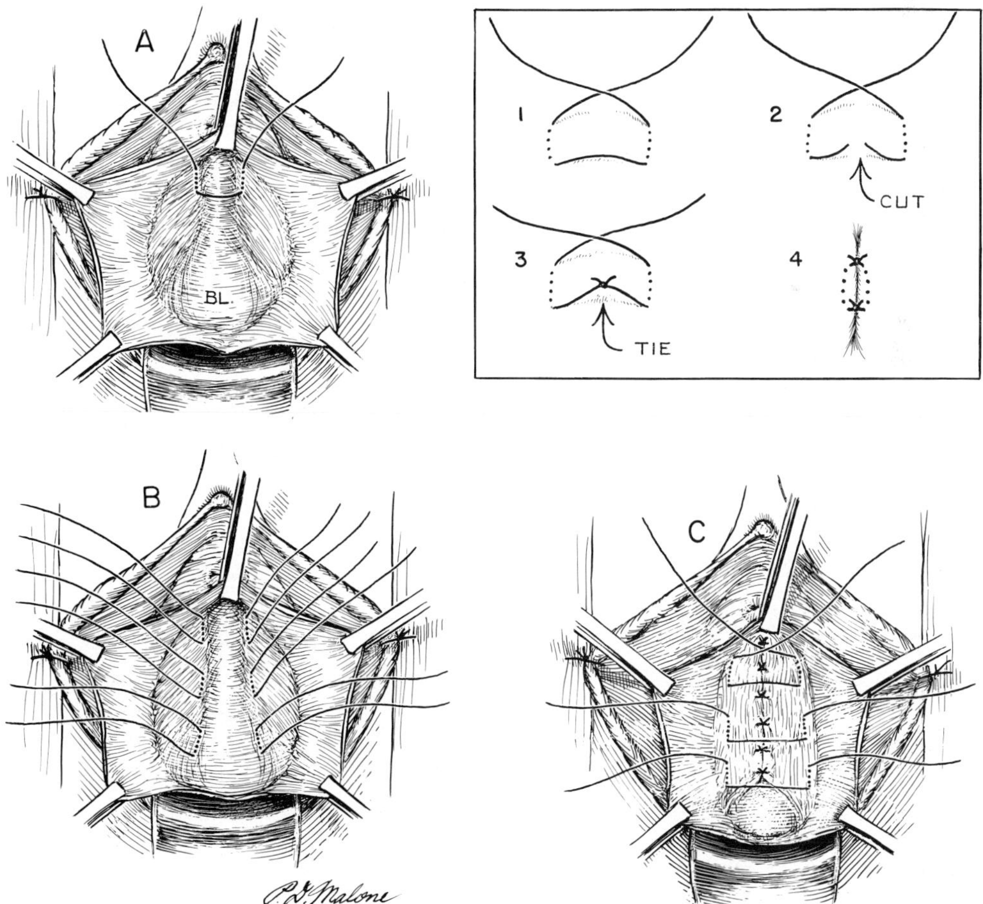

Figure 40. *A* through *C,* Double plication of vesicourethral angle utilizing the modified twin stitch of Tauber (1 through 4, *inset*), followed by a second row of plicating sutures.

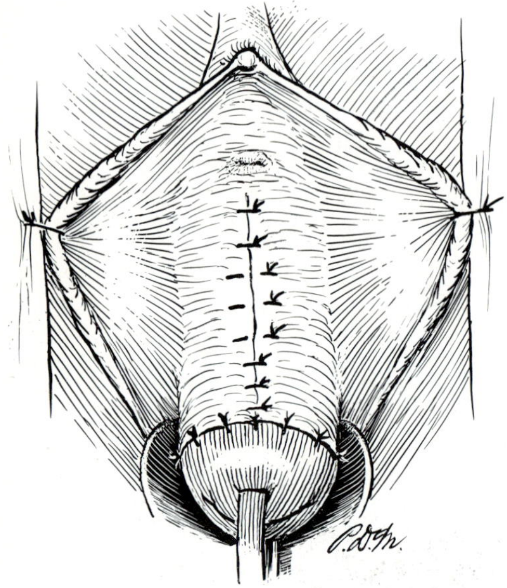

Figure 41. Double plication of vesicourethral angle. Redundant mucosa has been excised and the mucosa approximated. Vertical mattress sutures are placed through the mucosa beneath the vesicourethral angle.

Pubococcygeoplasty (Modified Ingelman-Sundberg Procedure)

Technique. A cervical mucosal incision is made from one lateral midpoint of the introitus to the other, with the apex of the incision 1 cm proximal to the external urethral orifice (Fig. 42). The mucosa is carefully freed from the underlying urethra and bladder base. A single layer of plicating sutures is placed beneath the urethra and bladder neck (see previous section). A Kelly clamp is employed to mobilize a segment of fascia and muscle beneath the pubic ramus (Fig. 43). This segment is then divided as low as possible so that the anterior segment on each side may be approximated with 1–0 chromic catgut or polyglycolic acid sutures in the midline beneath the vesicourethral angle without too much tension (Fig. 44). The same sutures used to approximate the muscle and fascia are (after tying) brought through the mucosa to anchor it to the operative site. A narrow rim of excess mucosa is trimmed before closure of the mucosa with interrupted 3–0 polyglycolic acid sutures (Fig. 45). An opening is made at the base of the mucosa for drainage because the operative site is quite vascular. A tight pack is placed in the vagina, and a suprapubic catheter is inserted.

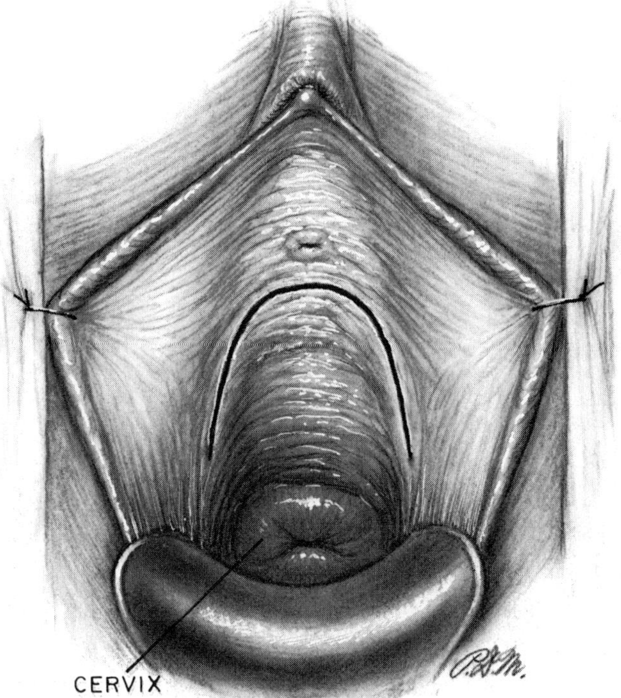

Figure 42. Pubococcygeoplasty. Mucosal incision extends from the lateral borders of the introitus to a point 1 cm behind the urethral orifice. (From Copenhaver, EH: Pubococcygeoplasty in the treatment of stress incontinence of urine. Lahey Clin Found Bull 27:58, April-June, 1978.)

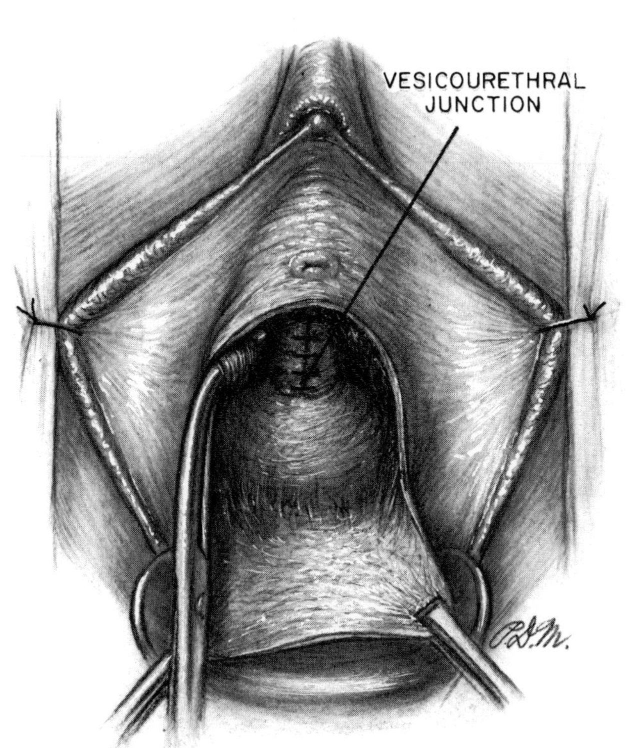

Figure 43. Pubococcygeoplasty. A segment of pubococcygeal muscle with fascia, 1 to 1.5 cm wide, is undermined and mobilized with a Kelly clamp after plicating sutures have been placed beneath the proximal urethra and bladder neck. (From Copenhaver, EH: Pubococcygeoplasty in the treatment of stress incontinence of urine. Lahey Clin Found Bull 27:59, April-June, 1978.)

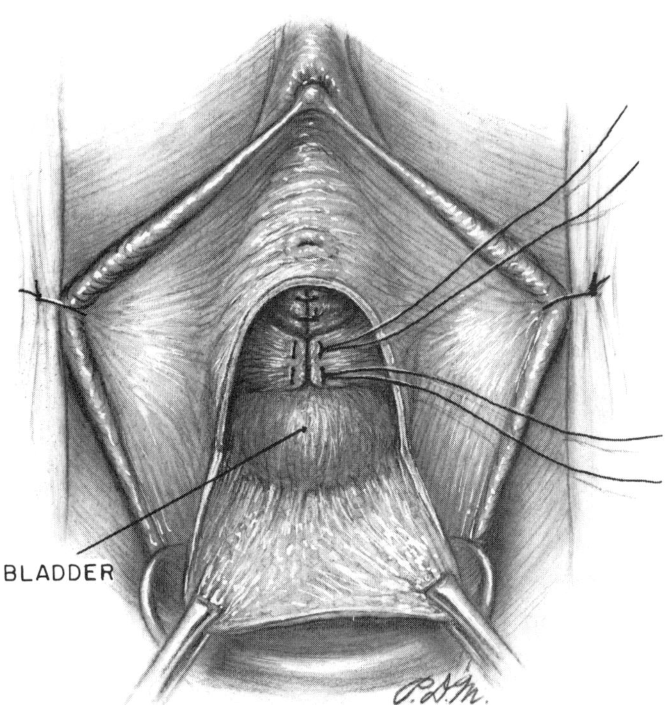

Figure 44. Pubococcygeoplasty. The muscle sling has been divided, and its anterior segments are approximated beneath the vesicourethral angle. (From Copenhaver, EH: Pubococcygeoplasty in the treatment of stress incontinence of urine. Lahey Clin Found Bull 27:59, April-June, 1978.)

Figure 45. Pubococcygeoplasty. A small buttonhole has been made in the deep base of the mucosal flap to permit drainage. The previous midline sutures have been brought through the mucosa to close the dead space. Redundant mucosa has been excised and the mucosa has been reapproximated. (From Copenhaver, EH: Pubococcygeoplasty in the treatment of stress incontinence of urine. Lahey Clin Found Bull 27:60, April-June, 1978.)

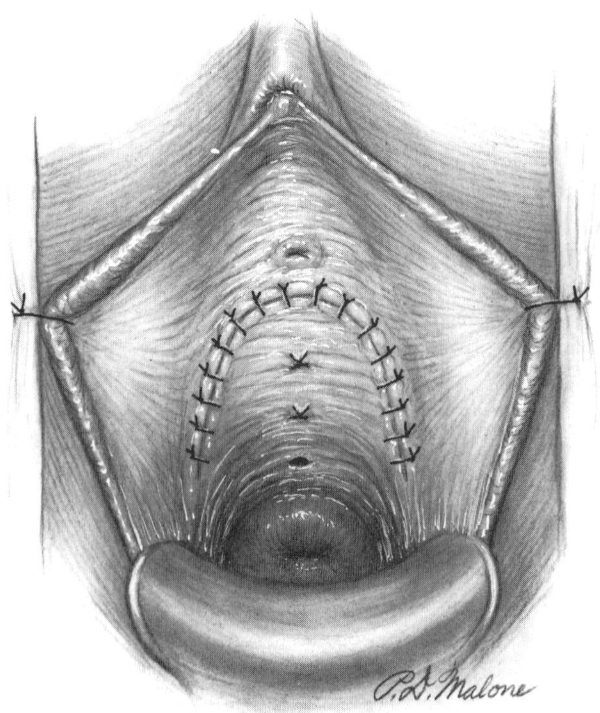

Sling Procedure

Technique. Manufactured materials have not been used successfully as a sling. Therefore, the sling should be obtained from the fascia lata. A strip, 18 cm × 0.5 cm to 1 cm, should be obtained. For the fascia lata a transverse incision, 5 cm, should be made 5 cm above the lateral condyle of the femur and carried down to the fascia where the fascia is cleared and undermined first toward the knee for several centimeters and then up the lateral midline of the leg until the desired length is obtained; a Masson fascia stripper may be used. The fascial defect need not be closed; the skin is approximated with vertical mattress 3–0 silk sutures, and a tight dressing is placed on the leg to cover the entire area of dissection.

At the outset a combined abdominal and vaginal preparation and draping should be carried out. The bladder should be emptied. A short anterior midline vaginal mucosal incision should be made beneath the urethra and bladder; the mucosa should be undermined so that the vesicourethral angle is visualized clearly; lateral space should exist at the junction of the urethra and bladder to permit the passing of a clamp. A low transverse incision, 5 cm, is made in the abdomen down to the fascia. A small vertical incison is made through the midline of the fascia. The retropubic space is entered easily through this incision and mobilized with a finger (Fig. 46). A long Kelly clamp is used to penetrate the rectus fascia 1 cm out from the midline above the symphysis pubis. The clamp is carefully passed behind the pubis with one hand, while the forefinger of the opposite hand is pushing upward through the vagina on the tissue lateral to the vesicourethral angle. Normal proprioceptive sensation makes this step relatively easy, and the clamp is thrust through the thin layer of tissue separating the retropubic space from the vagina. One end of the fascial strip is pulled upward and into view where it is sutured with 2–0 silk to the rectus fascia. The long Kelly clamp is pushed through to the vagina lateral to the opposite side of the vesicourethral angle, and the remaining end of the fascial strip is pulled upward and into view (Fig. 47). At this point enough tension is placed on the fascial strip to permit restitution of a normal vesicourethral angle. The master gynecologic surgeon, Richard W. Te Linde, would tap a glass catheter into the urethra and bladder with just slight resistance to test the desired and proper tension; the glass catheter has been replaced by a No. 10 French rubber catheter, but the concept is the same. While this correct degree of tension is maintained, the remaining end of the fascial strip is anchored to the rectus fascia. The short vertical midline incision is closed with 2–0 silk sutures, a suprapubic catheter is inserted into a bladder distended with saline solution, the abdominal wound is closed, and the vaginal incision is closed.

Postoperative Considerations. The patient is allowed to ambulate and have a regular diet as tolerated on the day after operation. A trial of voiding with the catheter open is held on the fourth postoperative day and with the catheter closed on the fifth postoperative day. Urinary retention is more common after the sling procedure. If retention occurs, the suprapubic catheter should not be removed until the patient has been able to void satisfactorily with low residual urine for two or three days. If the patient is unable to void and lives at a reasonable distance from the hospital, she may be discharged with instructions to close the catheter during the daytime at home and to open the stopcock when she is uncomfortable or for measurement of residual urine. She must be seen at weekly intervals and be instructed to come in immediately if the catheter becomes obstructed.

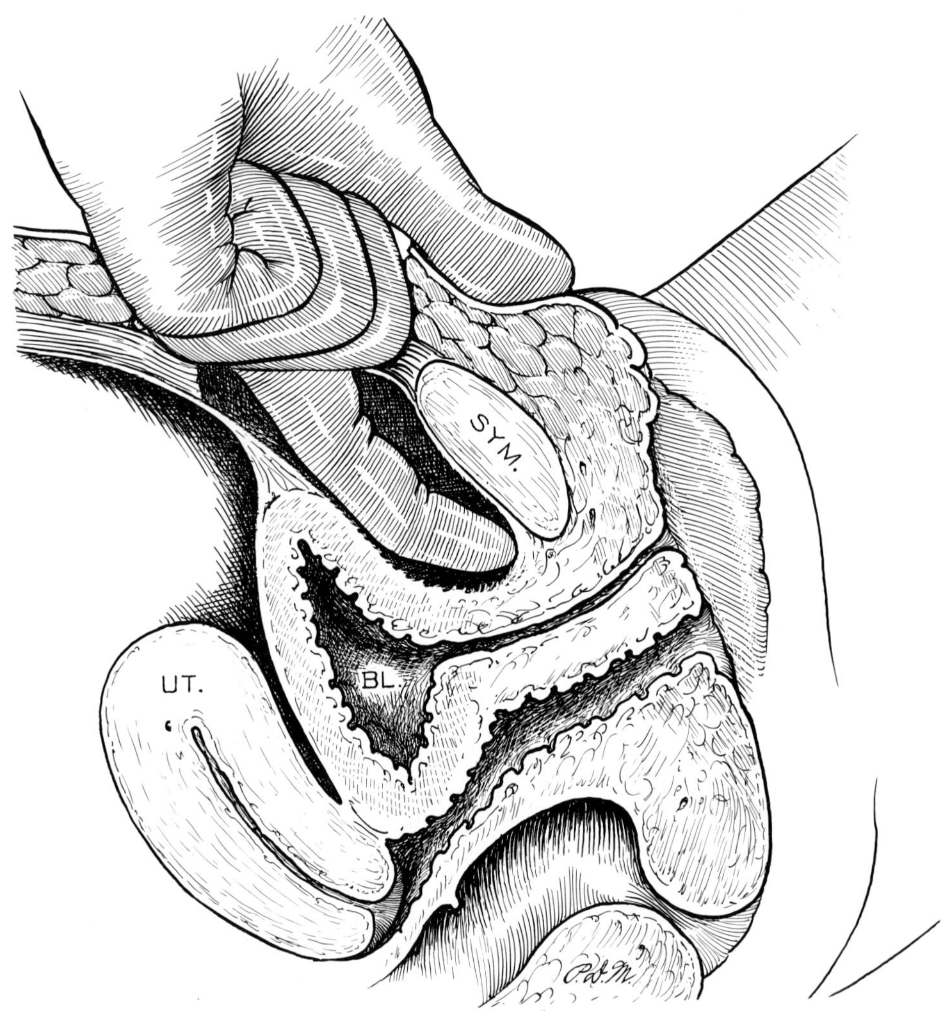

Figure 46.   Sling procedure. A small vertical midline incision has been made through the fascia to permit the forefinger to mobilize the retropubic space.

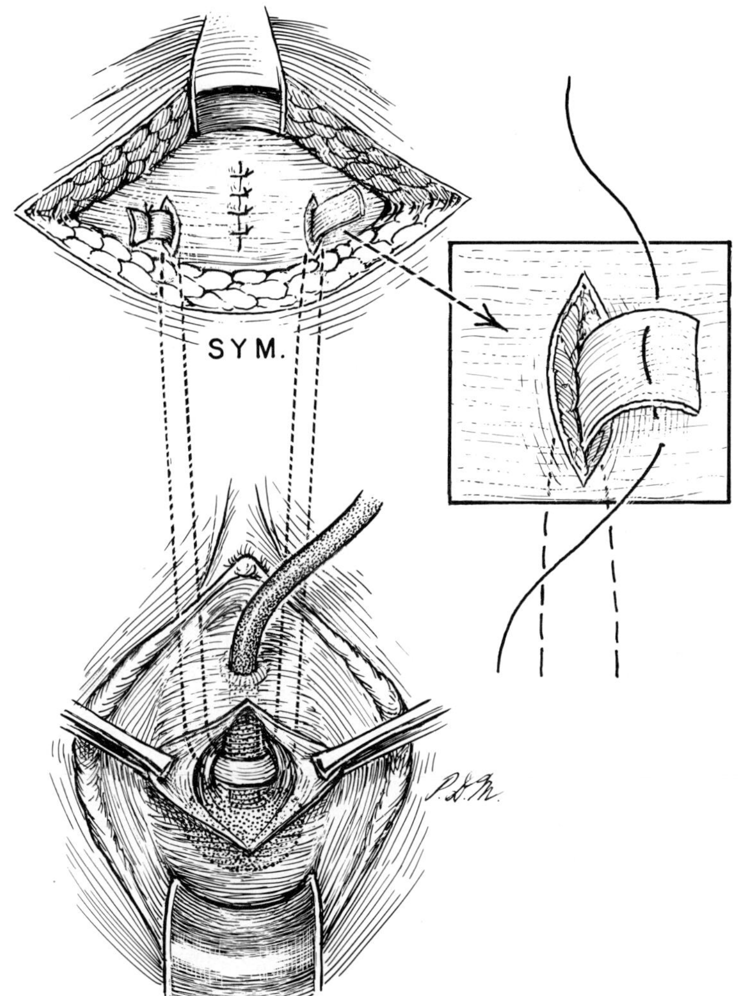

Figure 47. Sling procedure. A sling of fascia lata has been placed around the vesicourethral angle and is anchored to the rectus fascia with silk sutures.

VAGINAL MYOMECTOMY

Comments. A leiomyoma may arise from the cervix or from the uterine fundus and be visible or palpable on office examination or when curettage is performed. If a leiomyoma is found during the office examination, the patient should be admitted to the hospital for examination and treatment under anesthesia. The patient should be prepared as for major surgery.

Technique. If the leiomyoma arises from the fundus and is connected by a narrow stalk, multiple twisting will permit a simple removal. If the stalk will not allow turning of the tumor with ease, a 1–0 chromic catgut tie should be placed around the stalk to facilitate shelling out the tumor distal to the ligature. Should a leiomyoma be attached firmly within the uterine cavity, the preferred approach would be via the abdomen rather than through a deep incision in the uterus, except when a vaginal hysterectomy is contemplated. Two forms of cervical leiomyomas are approached vaginally — those arising from the endocervix when they could be shelled out easily and the vascular bed closed with a continuous suture, and those arising from the anterior surface beneath the bladder when the vesicouterine space could be opened easily, the superficial tumor removed, and the defect closed. In summary, only these simple myomectomies should be approached vaginally.

Postoperative Considerations. The patient may be managed as if minor surgery had been performed. No pack or catheter is used. However, the physician should be alert to delayed bleeding and infection, particularly when a leiomyoma has been removed by twisting or ligature of its stalk. In the latter instances it would be wise to observe the patient for several days in the hospital, unless she lives nearby. Also, if necrosis or infarction was evident at the time of operation, prophylactic antibiotics should be employed.

VAGINAL HYSTERECTOMY

Comments. If vaginal hysterectomies were performed only for absolute indications, few such operations would be done. Hysterectomy is an extension of the treatment of uterine prolapse. In most instances of intractable uterine bleeding, hysterectomy is viewed as elimination of an unpleasant nuisance rather than as a life-saving measure. The vaginal hysterectomy, when technically feasible, is the procedure of choice when treating a problem that requires removal of the uterus in a young woman who has completed childbearing. Use of this procedure could be restricted to those patients with small, symptomatic uterine leiomyomas and those with carcinoma in situ of the cervix. Of course, even these indications may be challenged, for a conservative operation may suffice. The liberal trend toward vaginal hysterectomy seems to be a conscious or unconscious effort on the part of some physicians and patients to improve a woman's "quality of life" by ridding her of menstrual problems and perhaps, secondarily, of the fear of pregnancy. With the present improvements in contraception and in sterilization techniques, perhaps this view should be tempered and the incidence of the operation reduced. Conversely, it might be argued that women with hypermenorrhea and dysmenorrhea have a right to be relieved of incapacitating symptoms rather than have to wait for menopause to provide a natural solution.

Currently, a candidate for simple vaginal hysterectomy has a preoperative evaluation on the morning of admission, undergoes operation in the afternoon, and is discharged on the third postoperative day — a three-day hospital stay.

Technique. Good instruments facilitate the vaginal hysterectomy. A long weighted vaginal retractor (Steiner), a Heaney retractor, a small Richardson retractor, two Heaney clamps, and two Heaney diamond jaw needle holders should be available. A suction tube is used. Two assistants are preferred.

The findings on pelvic examination should always be checked under anesthesia to confirm the feasibility of the vaginal approach, the uterus should be mobile and of reasonable size, the cul-de-sac should be free, and no evidence of adnexal disease should be present. If a vaginal repair is to be performed, both the genital area and the lower abdomen should be prepared and draped. A sterile sheet is tucked under the patient, and an adherent plastic drape is used to cover the buttocks and anal area. The bladder should be emptied with a straight catheter.

The uterine cavity is sounded, the cervix is dilated, and a routine curettage is performed. If any abnormal tissue is obtained, frozen section is requested before proceeding further. If carcinoma in situ of the cervix has not been defined precisely, a cone of the cervix is given to the pathologist for immediate examination.

Redundant labia minora are sutured to the drape and a 1 to 200,000 solution of epinephrine may be injected beneath the mucosa around the base of the cervix (Fig. 48). A circumscribing incision is made around the base of the cervix (or 2 cm beyond any area not stained with Schiller's solution in the case of carcinoma in situ of the cervix), and the mucosa is stripped back for 1.5 cm with Metzenbaum scissors. The cervix is pulled upward, the peritoneum of the cul-de-sac placed on tension, and the cul-de-sac is entered through a short, sharp incision with the scissors (Fig. 49). The adnexa are palpated, the long weighted retractor is placed in the cul-de-sac, and a long sponge is placed in the pelvis over the retractor to provide exposure. The patient is placed in the Trendelenburg position. The space between the cervix and bladder floor is opened by sharp dissection with the scissors (Fig. 50), and the vesicouterine peritoneum is grasped with Allis clamps and incised with scissors (Fig. 51 *A*). If entry is difficult beneath the bladder, it is best to proceed with the hysterectomy and to identify the bladder and vesicouterine peritoneum with a forefinger before incision (Fig. 51 *B*). This maneuver is especially applicable when the patient has had a previous low cesarean section. The

paracervical tissue and uterine vessels are systematically divided and ligated with No. 1 chromic catgut sutures (Figs. 52 through 54). If morcellation of the uterus is required, incisions are begun above the uterine vessels and carried obliquely toward the dome of the fundus (Fig. 55). Do not cut through the fundus, but leave an attachment so that the cornu with the adnexa will fall medially as the cervix and midportion of the uterus are pulled downward. With or without morcellation, the round and ovarian ligaments with tube are clamped (Fig. 56), divided, and doubly ligated; the second ligature on each side is held with a Kelly clamp. If it seems advisable to remove the adnexa and they can be mobilized, the tube and ovary should be grasped with a long Babcock clamp and the infundibulopelvic ligament clamped with a single Heaney clamp, divided, and doubly ligated with free No. 1 chromic catgut ties. When a segment of an ovary is to be removed, it is wise to start the running catgut suture (Ethicon G123 chromic catgut 2–0) before making the incision and to reinforce the closure with a separate figure-of-eight suture with 2–0 chromic catgut. If an enterocele is present, it is corrected by excising the redundant peritoneum (Fig. 57). McCall's suture technique has been abandoned. At this point the 1–0 suture (Davis & Geck TT3 Dexon 1–0 or Ethicon U246 chromic catgut 1–0) is used for the angle-supporting suture, starting with the lateral angle of the apical vaginal mucosa, picking up an edge of peritoneum and the previously ligated ligaments, and returning back through the mucosa. Tying the angle sutures and holding them with straight clamps facilitates placement of the peritoneal closure sutures (Fig. 58). The peritoneal closure (Davis & Geck TT3 Dexon 1–0 or Ethicon U246 chromic catgut 1–0) is begun on the patient's right side with a 1 cm edge of posterior peritoneum, the stumps of the ligated round and ovarian ligaments, and a 1 cm edge of anterior peritoneum (Fig. 59 *A*). This suture is tied, making certain that any previously ligated tissue is extraperitonealized. One end of the suture is held with a Kelly clamp as the previous ligature identified with a Kelly clamp is cut on that side. A similar suture is placed, starting with the patient's left anterior peritoneum, tied, and run as a continuous suture, extending to the peritoneal suture on the patient's right side (Fig. 59 *B*). When the peritoneum is closed, the continuous suture is tied to the previously placed right peritoneal suture and cut. The angle sutures held with straight clamps are placed on tension to permit transverse closure of the vagina with simple, figure-of-eight, or vertical mattress sutures (Davis & Geck TT3 Dexon 1–0 or Ethicon U246 chromic catgut 1–0). Any oozing tissue is sutured superficially with the mucosa to provide hemostasis and to close the dead space (Fig. 60). If a repair is to be accomplished, the middle third or half of the mucosa is left open as a starting point for an anterior or posterior repair. If an anterior repair alone is to be carried out, the redundant midline posterior mucosa may be closed vertically with a figure-of-eight suture (Davis & Geck TT3 Dexon 1–0 or Ethicon U246 chromic catgut 1–0). Oozing of blood above the vaginal apex unquestionably contributes to hematoma and infection of the vault, which are the causes of most febrile morbidity after vaginal hysterectomy. Tight closure, reduction of dead space, and use of a vaginal pack combined with prophylactic antibiotics are methods employed by the author, but it is acknowledged that leaving a vaginal mucosal defect, using a drain, using a suction catheter, and initial cauterization of the cervix are other logical ways to reduce morbidity. When no repair is performed a No. 14 5 cc Foley catheter is inserted, whereas a suprapubic catheter (Dow Cystocath No. 12) is used in the presence of a repair. A 2 inch gauze vaginal pack is inserted tightly into the vagina.

Postoperative Considerations. When vaginal hysterectomy alone has been performed, the Foley catheter is removed the morning after operation, and the patient is allowed out of bed as desired. The vaginal pack usually is removed two hours after operation but is retained overnight if operative bleeding was excessive. Prophylactic antibiotics are used. If suprapubic bladder drainage is employed, the patient is allowed to void on the fourth postoperative day (see section on vaginal repair). In the absence of repair, the patient is discharged on the third postoperative day if she is doing well.

Text continued on page 65.

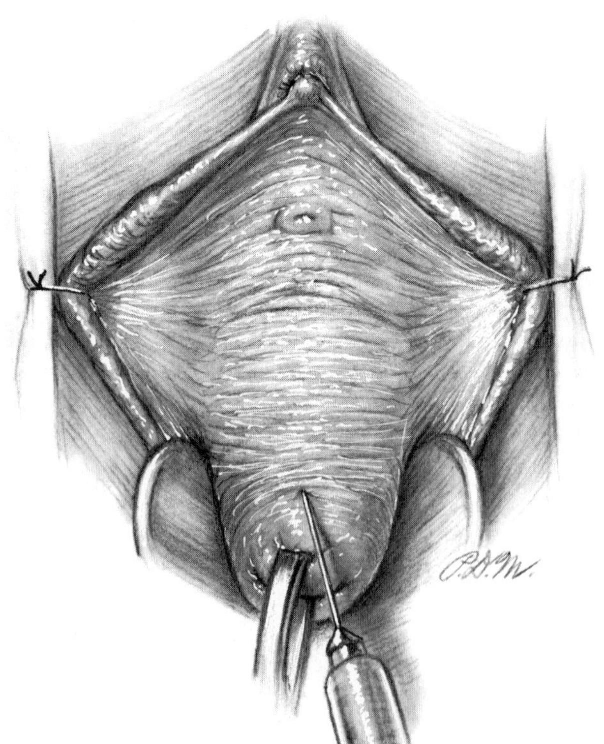

Figure 48. Vaginal hysterectomy. Redundant labia minora are sutured to the drape, and a 1 to 200,000 solution of epinephrine may be injected beneath the mucosa around the base of the cervix.

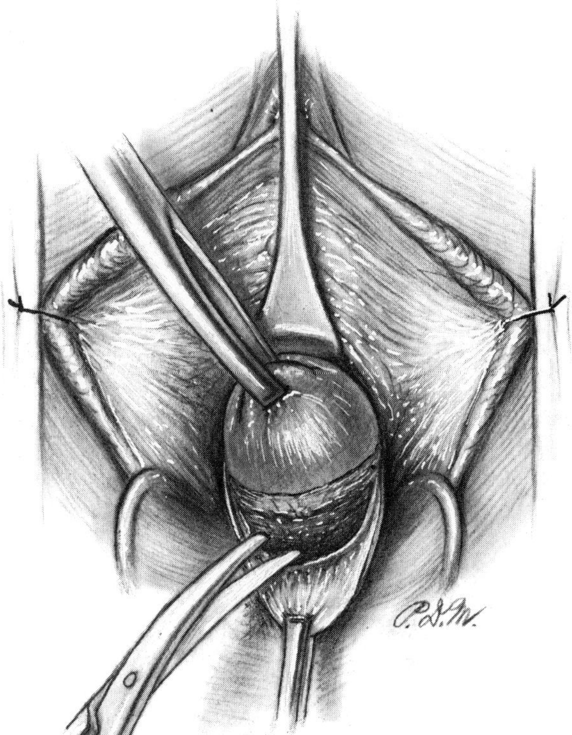

Figure 49.   Vaginal hysterectomy. Opening of the cul-de-sac.

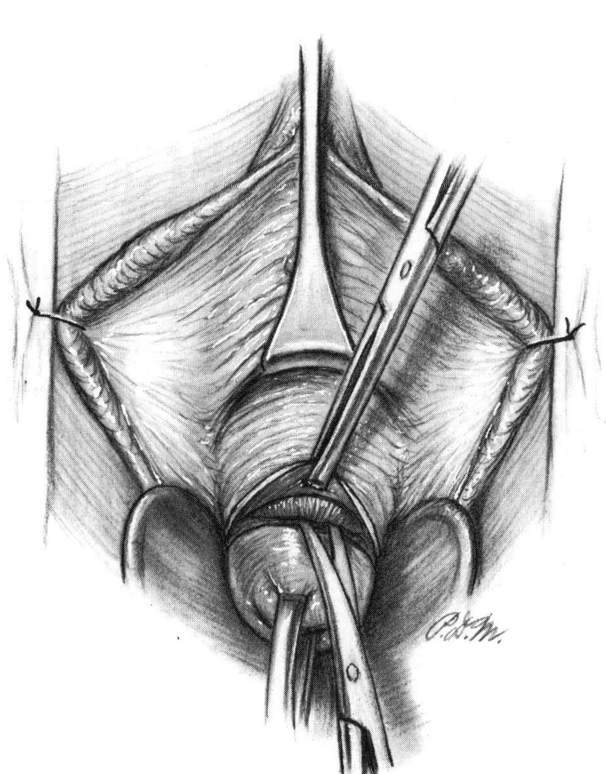

Figure 50.   Vaginal hysterectomy. Dissection of the space between the bladder and the cervix.

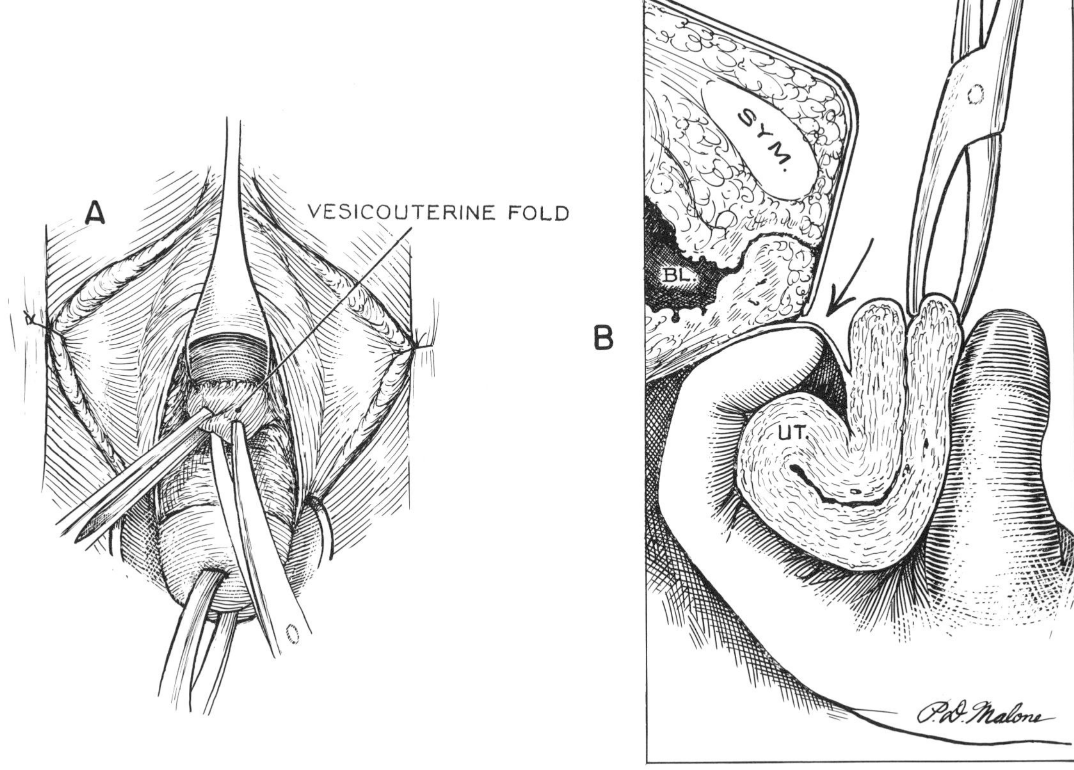

Figure 51. Vaginal hysterectomy. A and B, Alternative methods of identifying and incising the vesicouterine peritoneum.

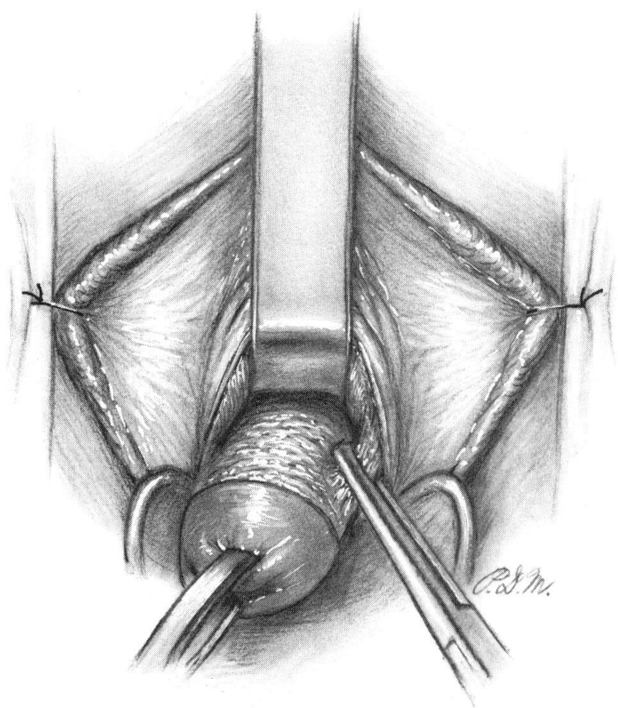

Figure 52. Vaginal hysterectomy. Clamping of paracervical tissues adjacent to the bladder.

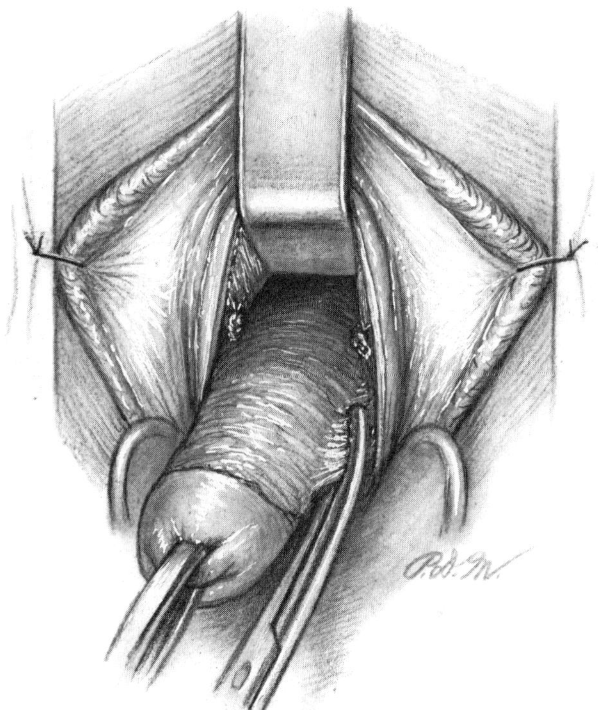

Figure 53. Vaginal hysterectomy. Clamping of the uterosacral ligament.

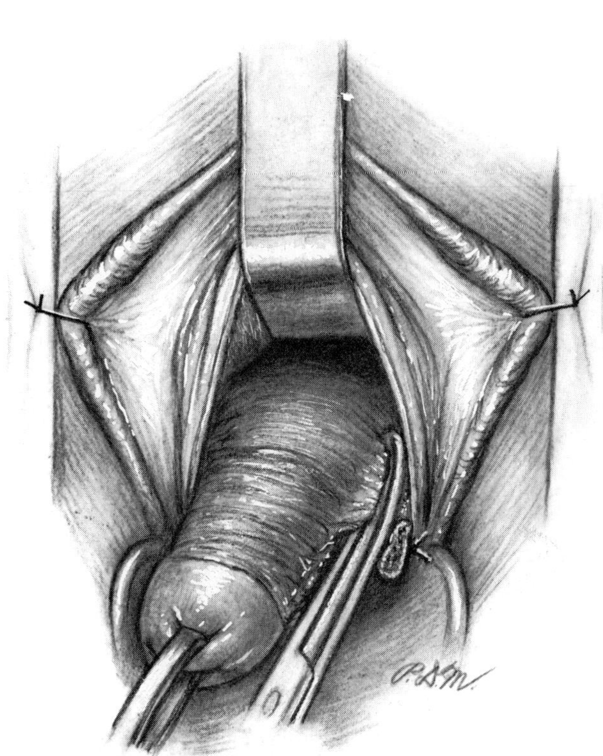

Figure 54. Vaginal hysterectomy. Clamping of the uterine vessels.

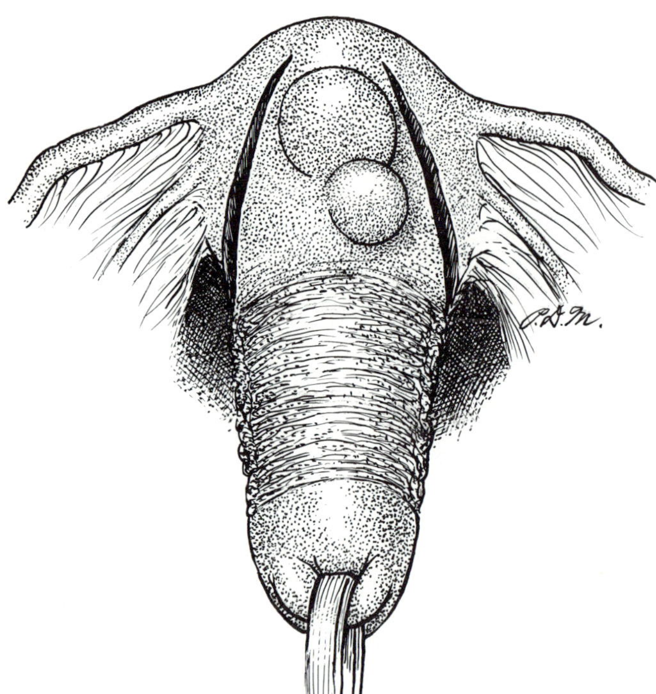

Figure 55. Vaginal hysterectomy. Wedge incision of the uterine fundus to permit removal of an enlarged uterus.

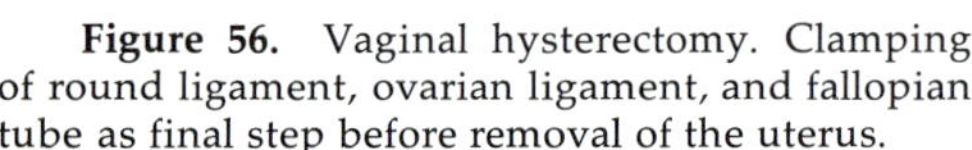

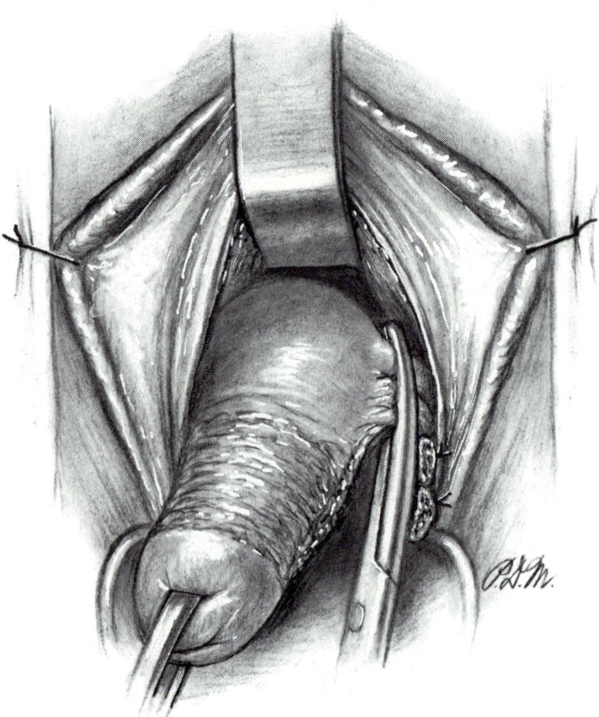

Figure 56. Vaginal hysterectomy. Clamping of round ligament, ovarian ligament, and fallopian tube as final step before removal of the uterus.

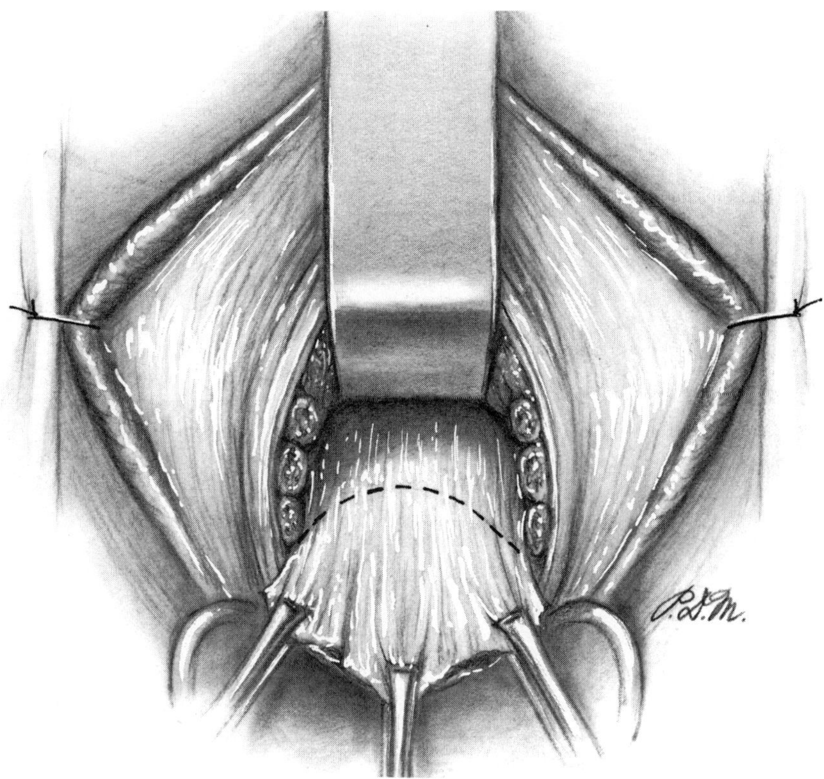

Figure 57. Vaginal hysterectomy. Excision of redundant peritoneum of enterocele.

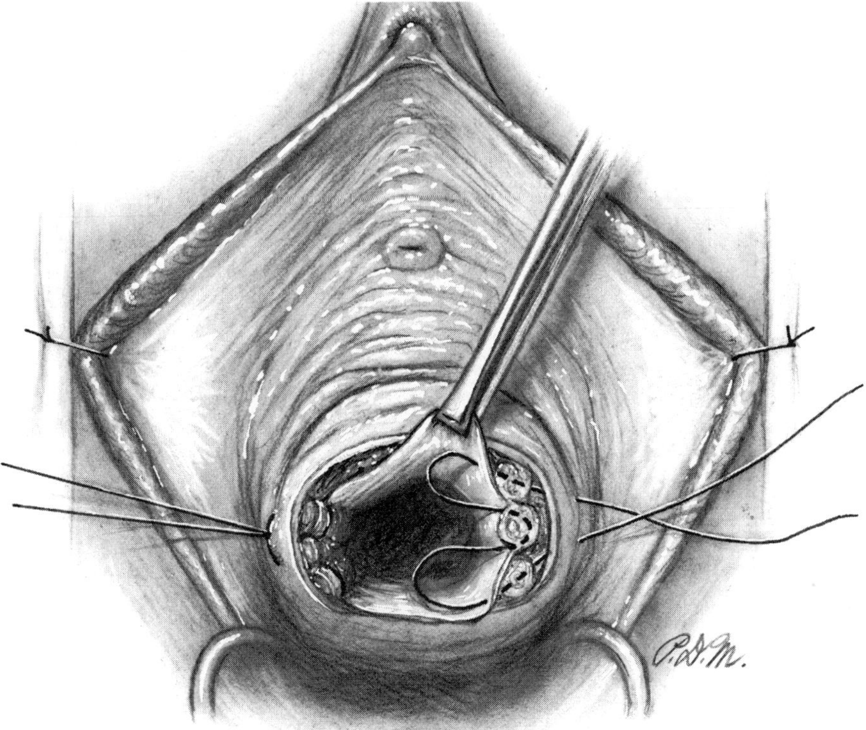

Figure 58. Vaginal hysterectomy. Anchoring ligaments and peritoneum to the lateral angles of the vagina.

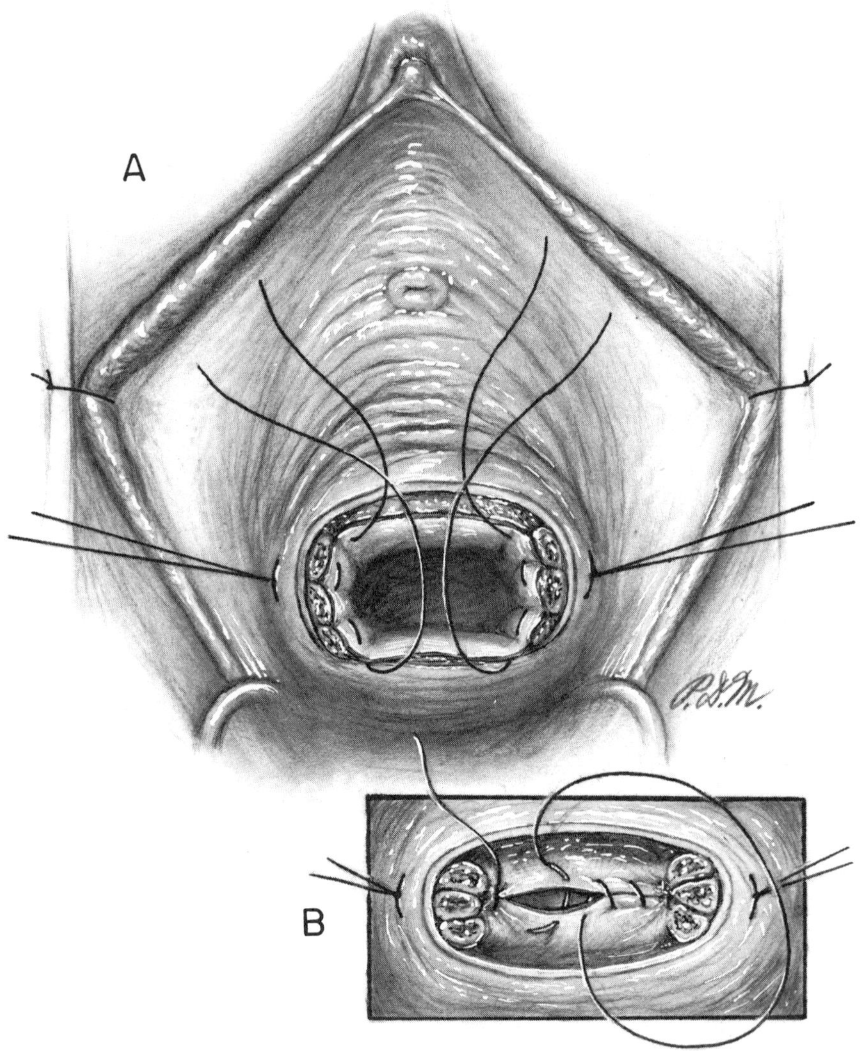

Figure 59. Vaginal hysterectomy. *A,* Closure of the peritoneal angle on the surgeon's left side followed by closure of the opposite angle and *B,* a precise peritoneal closure with a continuous suture, which is tied to the left peritoneal angle suture.

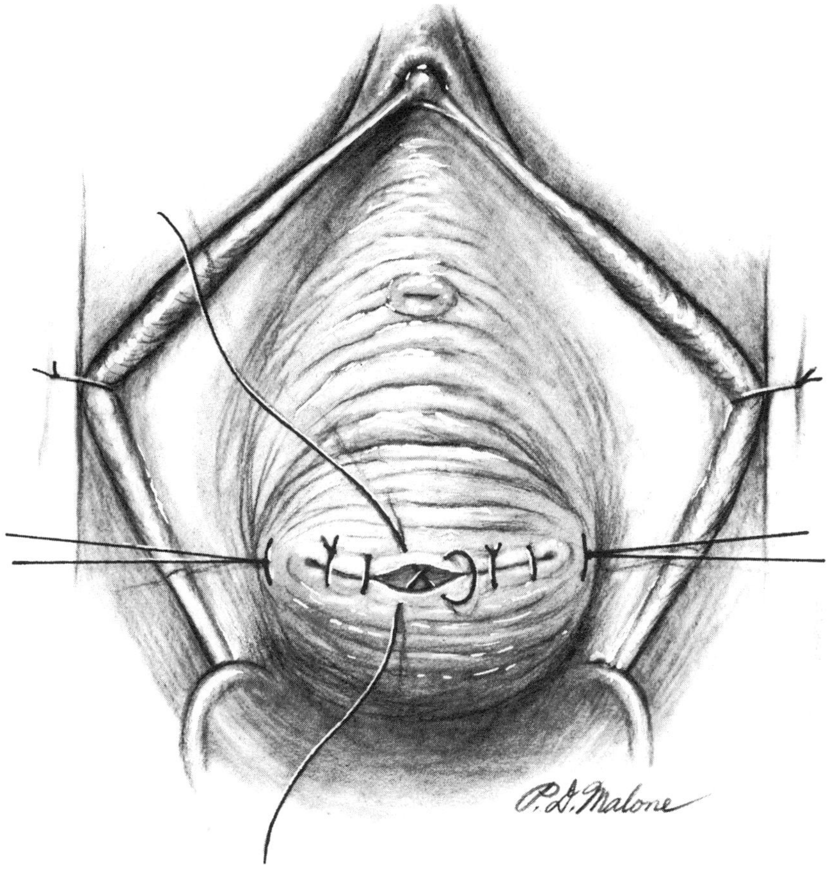

Figure 60. Vaginal hysterectomy. Transverse closure with figure-of-eight sutures.

AMPUTATION OF THE CERVIX WITH REPAIR (MODIFIED MANCHESTER PROCEDURE)

Comments. Amputation of the cervix with repair is a good and sound operative procedure that should be used more frequently. This procedure is particularly applicable in postmenopausal women with prolapse of an elongated and enlarged uterus. It provides as good a result as vaginal hysterectomy but with less associated morbidity. On the other hand, it does not terminate childbearing and does not eliminate the uterine fundus as a future source of disease.

Technique. Preparation and draping of the patient are the same as for vaginal hysterectomy. Since an anterior vaginal repair is customarily performed, the lower abdomen is prepared for insertion of a suprapubic catheter. The bladder is emptied. Dilatation and curettage are performed. A circumscribing mucosal incision is made around the base of the cervix, and the mucosa is stripped back for a short distance. The space between the cervix and bladder is opened by sharp dissection, and the paracervical tissue adjacent to the bladder base and lateral angles of the cervix is divided and ligated with No. 1 chromic catgut sutures. Hemostatic No. 1 chromic catgut sutures on a cutting needle are placed deeply into each side of the cervix (Fig. 61). Any defect posterior to the cervix is repaired with pursestring and plicating sutures, the previously ligated stumps of paracervical tissue are attached to the upper anterior segment of cervix, 2 cm or more of cervix are amputated below the hemostatic sutures, and a Sturmdorf suture is employed to bring the posterior vaginal mucosa to the newly created cervical os. The anterior vaginal mucosa is undermined and incised, and a routine anterior vaginal repair is done (Fig. 62). Redundant anterior vaginal mucosa is excised (Fig. 63), and the mucosa is approximated with simple sutures (Davis & Geck TT3 Dexon 1–0). A special anterior version of the Sturmdorf suture is anchored to the anterior margin of the new cervical os (Fig. 64). Small mucosal defects remain on each side of the cervical os; they are closed with simple or figure-of-eight sutures (Fig. 65). A posterior vaginal repair is performed as necessary (see section on vaginal repair).

A vaginal gauze pack is inserted, saline solution, 400 cc, is instilled into the bladder, and a No. 12 Cystocath is inserted into the bladder for suprapubic drainage of urine.

Postoperative Considerations. Postoperative considerations are the same as those for vaginal hysterectomy or repair or both. The pack is removed in either two hours or the morning after operation, when the patient is allowed out of bed. A trial of voiding is begun on the fourth postoperative day, and the patient is discharged from the hospital about two days after a satisfactory voiding pattern has been established.

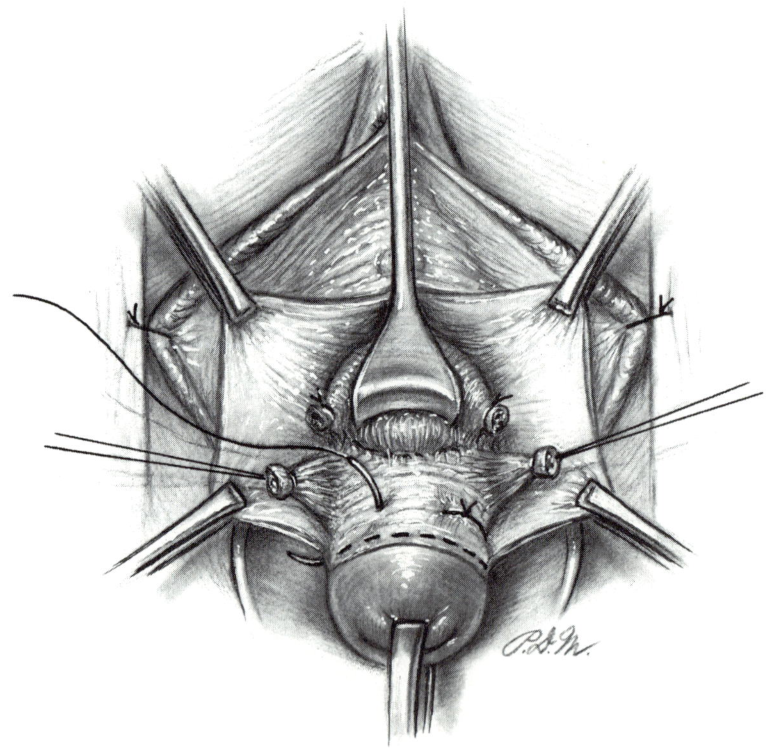

Figure 61. Amputation of the cervix with repair. A circumscribing incision has been made around the cervix, the base of the bladder has been separated from the cervix, and the paracervical tissue adjacent to the bladder base and at the lateral angles of the cervix has been divided and ligated. Hemostatic sutures are being placed deeply into each side of the cervix with a cutting needle.

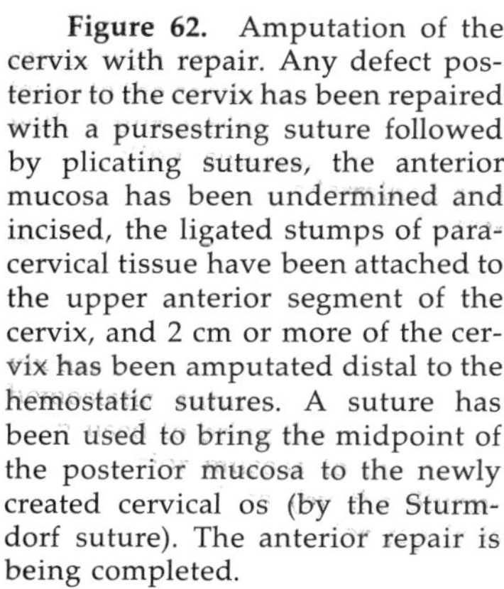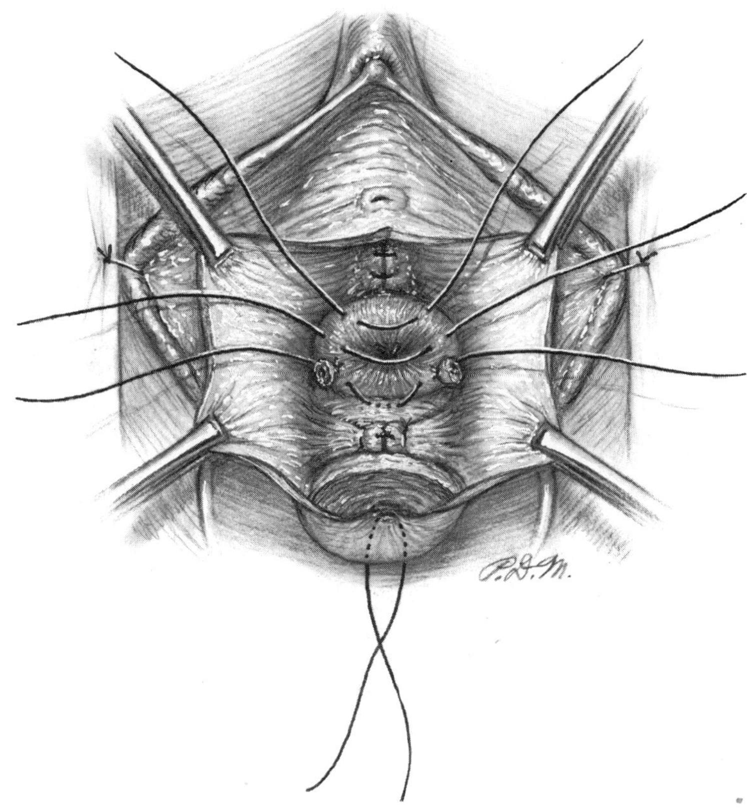

Figure 62. Amputation of the cervix with repair. Any defect posterior to the cervix has been repaired with a pursestring suture followed by plicating sutures, the anterior mucosa has been undermined and incised, the ligated stumps of paracervical tissue have been attached to the upper anterior segment of the cervix, and 2 cm or more of the cervix has been amputated distal to the hemostatic sutures. A suture has been used to bring the midpoint of the posterior mucosa to the newly created cervical os (by the Sturmdorf suture). The anterior repair is being completed.

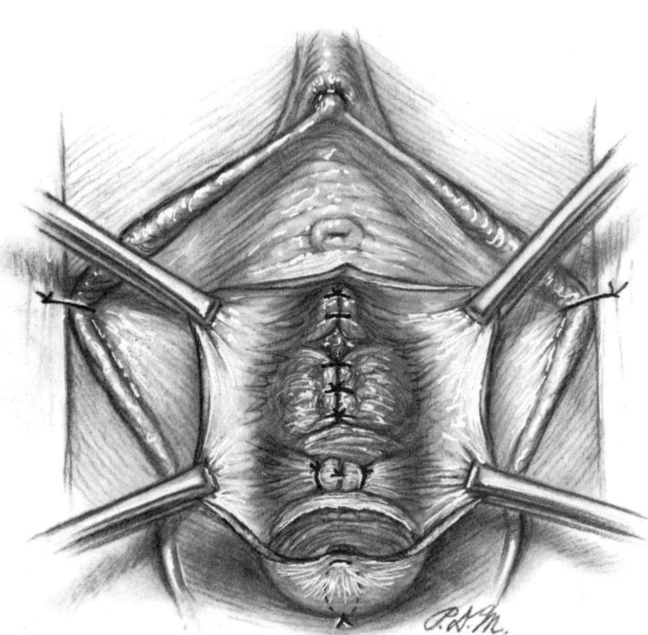

Figure 63. Amputation of the cervix with repair. The repair has been completed, and redundant mucosa has been excised.

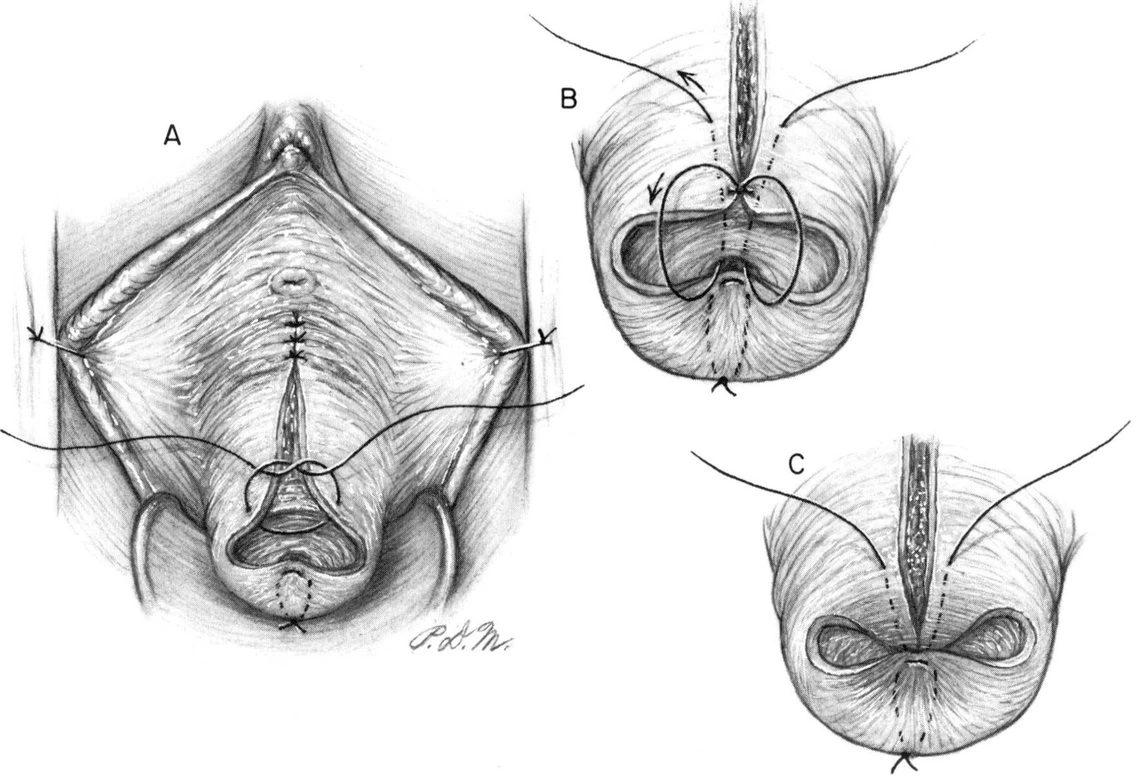

Figure 64. *A* through *C*, Amputation of the cervix with repair. The mucosa is approximated with simple sutures and with a special suture to attach the mucosa to the anterior cervical os.

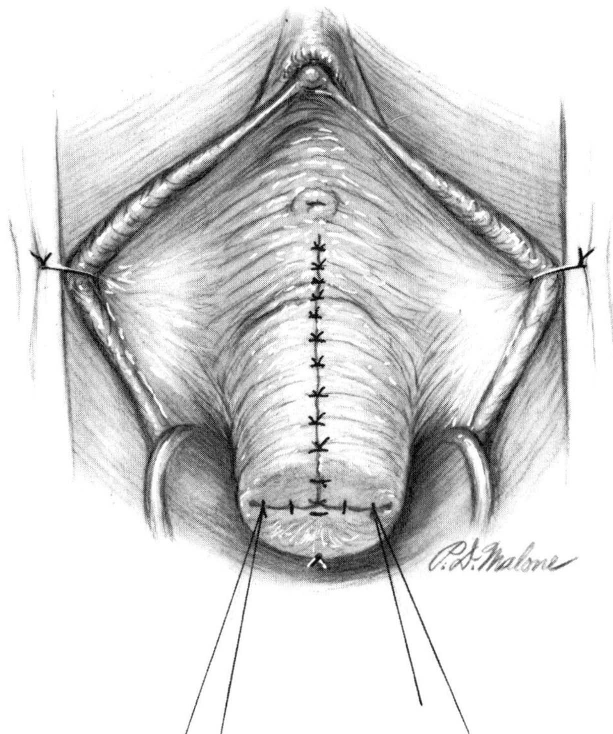

Figure 65. Amputation of the cervix with repair has been completed. The repair is shown everted for diagrammatic purposes.

VAGINAL REMOVAL OF CERVICAL STUMP

Comments.   Vaginal removal of a cervical stump has become a rare procedure because of the infrequency of subtotal hysterectomy. We use this procedure for carcinoma in situ and for symptomatic prolapse. In rare instances the cervical stump requires removal as part of a radical operation for invasive cancer. In this country, such a procedure is performed for the most part through the abdomen, and the same technique is used as for radical hysterectomy or exenteration. It should be added that therapeutic conization of the cervix would also be a consideration when dealing with carcinoma in situ in the cervical stump.

Technique.   The preparation and draping of the patient, emptying of the bladder, and sounding of the cervix are the same as for vaginal hysterectomy. A circumscribing mucosal incision should include a margin that is 2 cm beyond any carcinoma in situ or dysplasia as demonstrated by colposcopy or the Schiller test. The mucosa is stripped back over the cervix. It is not necessary to enter the peritoneal cavity; every bit of cervical stroma need not be removed. The paracervical tissue is divided and ligated with No. 1 chromic catgut sutures until the base of the stump is reached. Deep hemostatic sutures are then placed across the base of the cervical stump, and a subtotal removal is performed. Angle-supporting sutures are placed between the lateral angles of the vaginal mucosa and the previously ligated paracervical tissue. The vagina is closed transversely with simple or figure-of-eight sutures (Davis & Geck TT3 Dexon 1–0 or Ethicon U246 chromic catgut 1–0). If a repair is performed, the center portion of the apex is left open as a starting point for the repair. In the absence of repair, a vaginal pack and a No. 14 5 cc Foley catheter are inserted.

Postoperative Considerations.   In the absence of a repair the pack is removed in two hours, the catheter is removed the morning after operation, and the patient is discharged from the hospital on the second postoperative day. When a repair is performed, the postoperative management is the same as for repair alone (see section on vaginal repair).

REPAIR OF URINARY FISTULA

Comments.   At the Lahey Clinic fecal or intestinal fistulas are repaired by the proctologic surgeon, ureteral and bladder fistulas requiring an intraabdominal or intravesical approach by the urologic surgeon, and fistulas requiring only vaginal repair by the gynecologic surgeon. This approach places the patient in the most experienced hands for a particular problem.

To achieve success with any fistula repair, the surgeon must deal with tissues that are as healthy as possible. Therefore, a waiting period of six months between a bladder or urethral injury and the repair is advisable. With a fistula caused by irradiation, a period of observation is of special importance to determine the final extent and nature of the tissue breakdown and to assess whether viable tumor is involved in the process. While cortisone can accelerate the resolution of inflammation, the best results still follow the six-month waiting period. During the six months, the patient should use no tampons in the vagina, should not be catheterized, and should use no antibiotics. In the absence of natural estrogens, conjugated estrogens, 0.625 mg taken by mouth, should be prescribed for the first 25 days of each month, stopping one week before operation.

Simple Repair

Technique. A fine probe is inserted through the vaginal fistula into the bladder, and the vagina is packed with sponges. Cystoscopy is performed with a No. 22 or smaller Brown-Buerger cystoscope. The probe and fistula are easily visualized, and the relation of the ureteral orifices to the fistula is noted. If the ureteral orifices are close to the fistula site, No. 6 olive-tipped ureteral catheters are inserted into the ureters. The cystoscope is removed; then an incision, 1 cm, is made above the pubic symphysis, a long, narrow forceps (Randall kidney stone forceps, quarter curved) is inserted via the urethra through the dome of the distended bladder and suprapubic incision, and a No. 16 Silastic catheter with a bulb is pulled into the bladder to provide suprapubic bladder drainage. If the ureters require catheterization, a Foley catheter may be inserted into the urethra and the catheters tied securely to the Foley catheter with silk or catgut.

A No. 8 (or larger if necessary) Foley catheter is placed through the vagina into the fistula after removal of the probe and the vaginal sponges. This permits tension at the site of the fistula and thus better exposure. With tension on the catheter, a small scalpel blade is used first to circumscribe the vaginal opening of the fistula and then to circumscribe an area of vaginal mucosa 2 cm out from the opening (Fig. 66 *A*).* A fine suction tip is applied by the assistant to assure excellent exposure. The outlined circular area of thin vaginal mucosa is removed carefully in sections (Fig. 66 *B*).

With the Foley catheter remaining in the fistula and pulled to one side, a catgut suture on a delicate needle (Ethicon G123 chromic catgut 2–0) is placed at the lateral edge of the mucosal opening to the fistula. A simple running suture is continued as far as possible with the catheter in place (Fig. 67 *A*). If possible, the suture should be placed in the submucosa; however, if the tissue is too delicate, it should be placed through the mucosa.

The tension catheter is removed, and the fistula is closed in a transverse direction with a continuous suture. At this point normal saline solution, 200 cc, is instilled into the bladder via the suprapubic catheter to confirm closure to the fistula. The suture at each angle has been held to permit exposure and to begin a layer of interrupted plicating 2–0 chromic catgut sutures (Fig. 67 *B*). Each suture is tied and held with a clamp. If it is practical to place another layer of plicating sutures, do so and hold the sutures.

The posterior mucosa is mobilized by undermining for 1 cm, and a small needle is attached to the previously held sutures and placed through the lower portion of the undermined posterior flap of mucosa, thereby covering the fistula closure with healthy mucosa (Fig. 68 *A*). The remaining mucosa is approximated with single 2–0 or 3–0 polyglycolic acid sutures (Fig. 68 *B*).

If the vascularity of the tissue is poor, if the patient has previously undergone an unsuccessful repair, or if the patient has had previous irradiation, the mucosa should be approximated in a transverse direction with simple sutures of No. 26 silver wire. These sutures are not tied but twisted closed, and all are placed within rubber or plastic tubing, which is folded upon itself to remain in the vagina (Fig. 69 *A*). After two weeks (or more if the patient has had previous irradiation) and with the patient under anesthesia, *each* wire suture is carefully untwisted, and one end is cut close to the suture line. A right-angle clamp is placed loosely around the base of the other end of wire and the suture is gently removed (Fig. 69 *B*). An alternative to the use of wire would be to use 2–0 Tevdek sutures, leaving them in place for four weeks or more before careful removal in the office (or operating room, if necessary).

---

*Figures 66 through 72 were originally presented by the author as part of a talk, "Urethrovaginal and Vesicovaginal Fistula Repair — Transvaginal Approach," presented at the postgraduate education course on Pediatric and Adult Reconstructive Urologic Surgery, Boston, June 7, 1974.

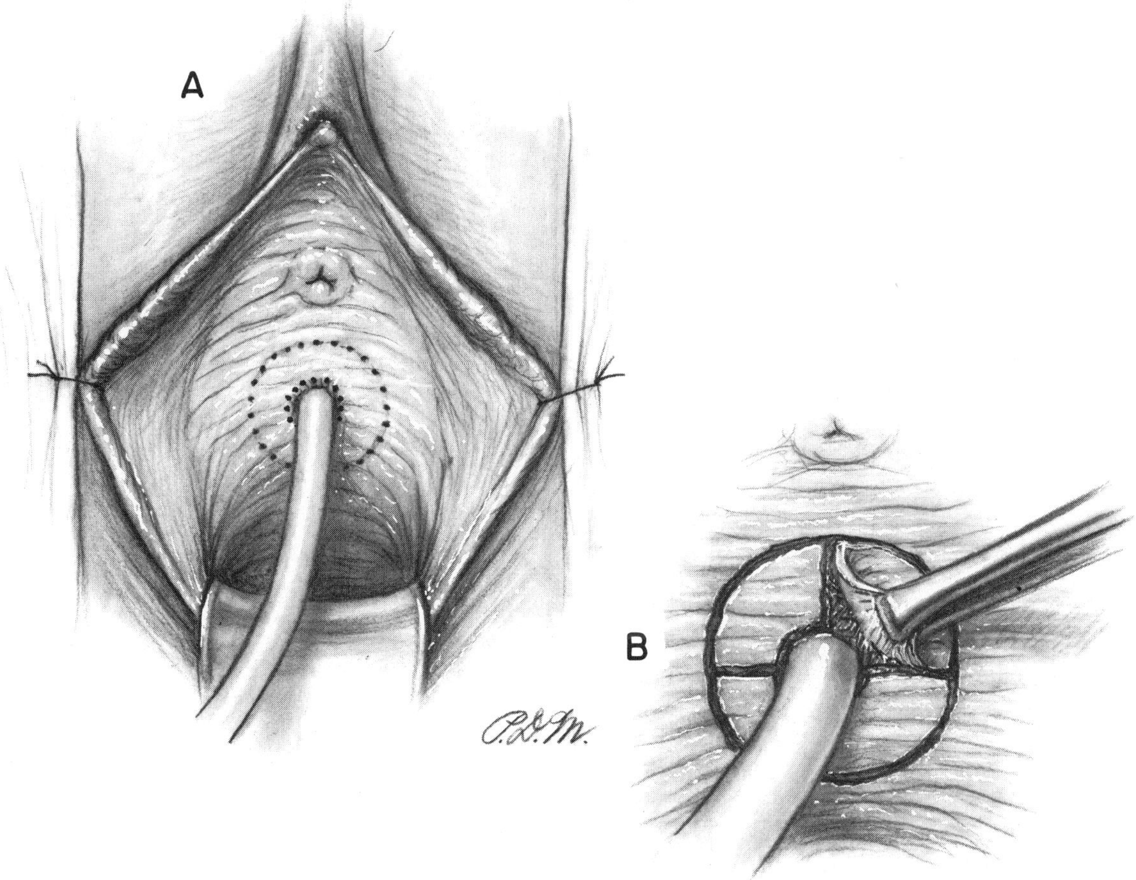

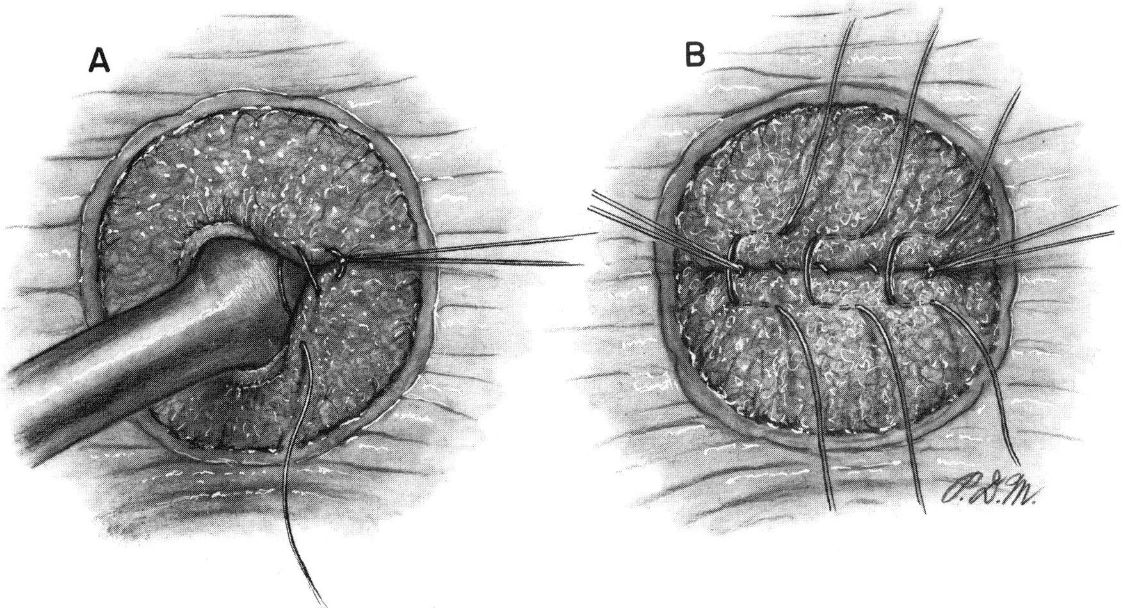

Figure 66. Repair of vesicovaginal fistula. *A,* A No. 8 Foley catheter has been placed through the fistula, tension placed on the catheter, and a circular area of mucosa is outlined for removal around the fistula. *B,* The mucosa is divided into quadrants to facilitate superficial removal.

Figure 67. Repair of vesicovaginal fistula. *A,* A continuous suture is begun at one angle of the fistula, avoiding the mucosa of the bladder or fistulous tract if possible. *B,* Plicating sutures are placed to reinforce the closure.

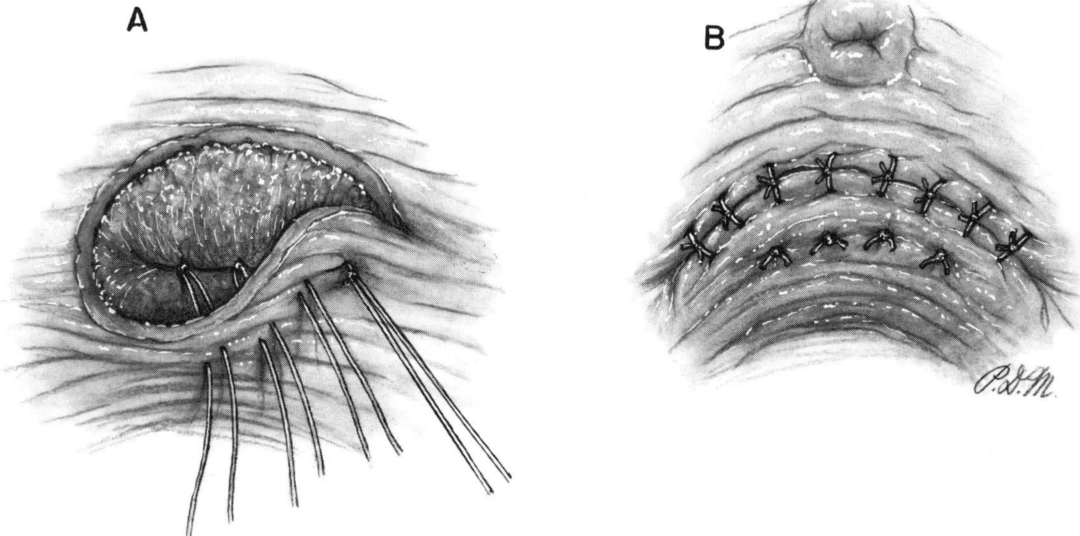

Figure 68.   Repair of vesicovaginal fistula. *A,* The tied plicating sutures are used to bring a slightly mobilized flap of posterior vaginal mucosa over the fistula repair. *B,* The mucosa is approximated with simple sutures.

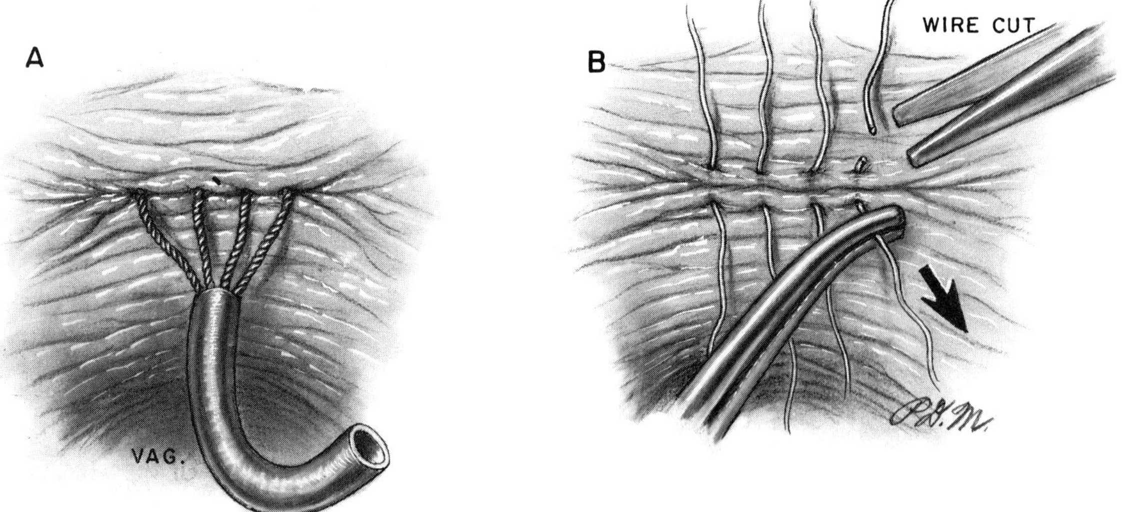

Figure 69.   Repair of vesicovaginal fistula. *A,* When a fistula has been resistant to repair in the past or when there is a history of irradiation, simple No. 26 silver wire sutures are used, twisted instead of tied, and placed within a rubber or plastic tube. *B,* After two or more weeks, the wire is untwisted and carefully cut close to the mucosal closure, avoiding the tearing of any tissue in the process.

Reconstruction of Urethra and Closure of Vesicovaginal Fistula

Technique. Cystoscopy and insertion of a suprapubic catheter are performed as described. A U-shaped incision is made, and the mucosa is mobilized to form a urethra 3 cm in length (Fig. 70 *A*). A Silastic splint is placed gently within the bladder and anchored to the vestibule or labium with 2–0 Tevdek sutures (Fig. 70 *B*). The urethra is constructed over the splint. At the base of the U, a continuous suture of 2–0 chromic catgut is placed (Fig. 71 *A*) and reinforced with interrupted plicating sutures (Fig. 71 *B*); the sutures are held. A flap of pubococcygeal muscle and fascia is mobilized from each side and approximated beneath the vesicourethral angle with a 1–0 chromic catgut suture (Fig. 72 *A*); the sutures are held. The vaginal mucosa is mobilized beneath the base of the bladder and attached to the reconstruction site with the previously held sutures. The remaining mucosal defects are closed with simple 2–0 or 3–0 polyglycolic acid sutures (Fig. 72 *B*).

Postoperative Considerations. Prophylactic antibiotics are given. The suprapubic catheter is irrigated with 0.25 per cent acetic acid, 25 cc, every six hours for 48 hours and as necessary thereafter. The suprapubic catheter is clamped, and the patient is permitted to void normally two weeks after simple closure of a small fistula and four weeks after closure of a large fistula or reconstruction of the urethra (the patient may be discharged after two weeks in the hospital, in the latter case with instructions for home catheter care and clamping). The clamp should be removed for discomfort, for measurement of residual urine at four-hour intervals, and during the night. A urethral splint may be removed after the patient is able to void around it. The suprapubic catheter is removed after one day of voiding in amounts of 100 cc or more and after repeated residual urines of less than 100 cc. Urine is obtained for culture before removal of the catheter. Nitrofurantoin (Furadantin), 100 mg by mouth every eight hours, is given until results of the urine culture are available.

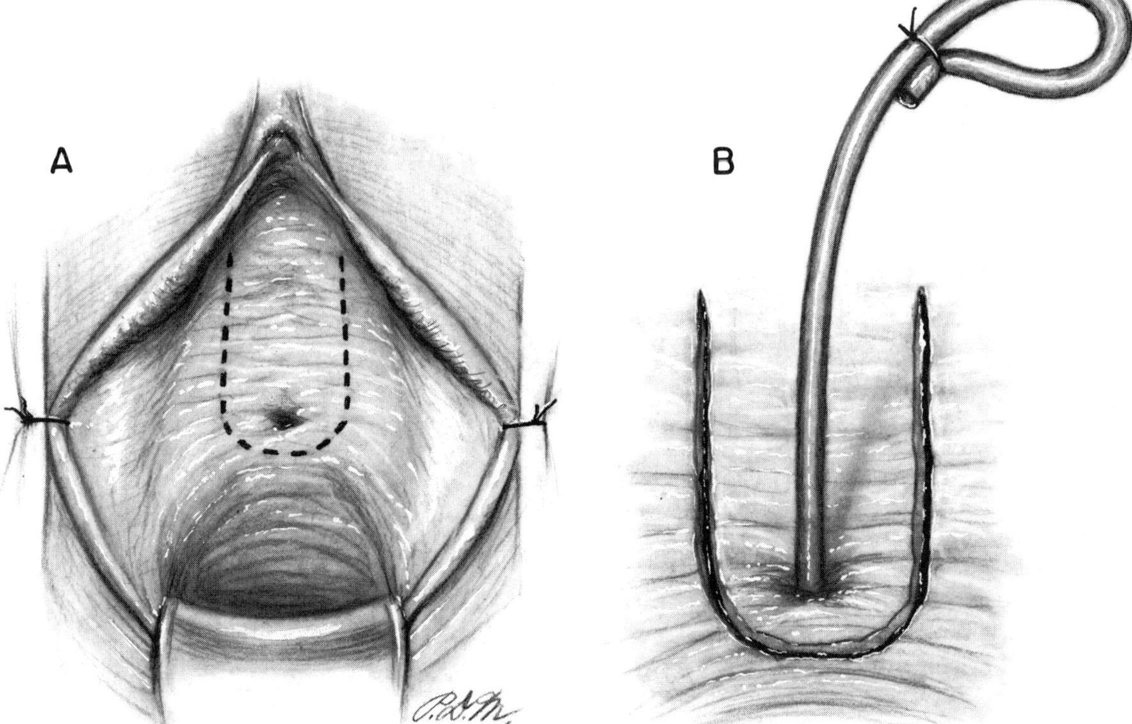

Figure 70.   Reconstruction of the urethra. *A,* A **U**-shaped mucosal incision outlines the new urethra. *B,* A Silastic tube is placed into the bladder and used as a splint for the new urethra.

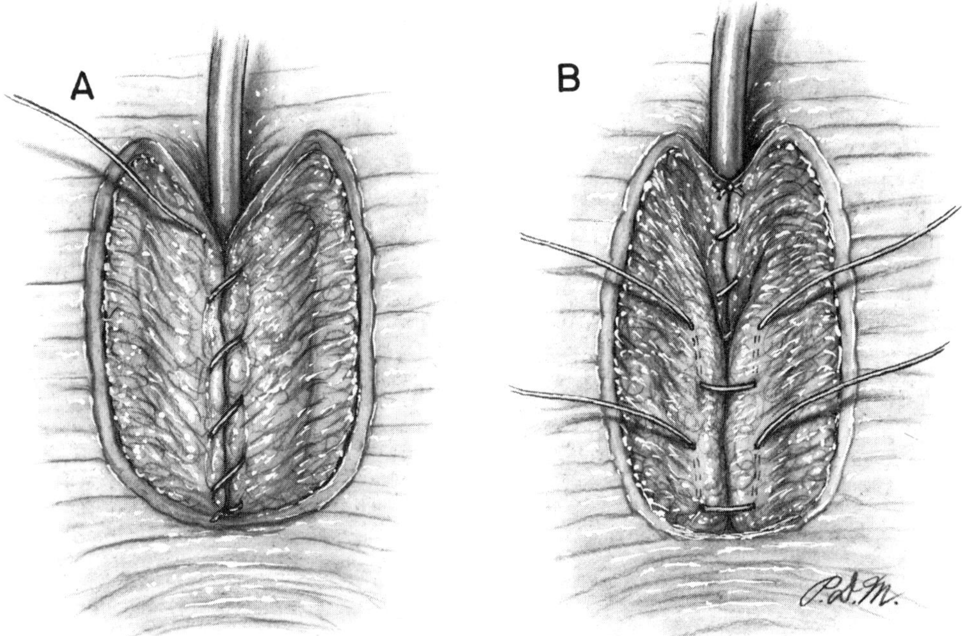

Figure 71.   Reconstruction of the urethra. *A,* A continuous suture is placed from the base of the **U** to the top of its lateral arms. *B,* Plicating sutures are placed to reinforce the closure.

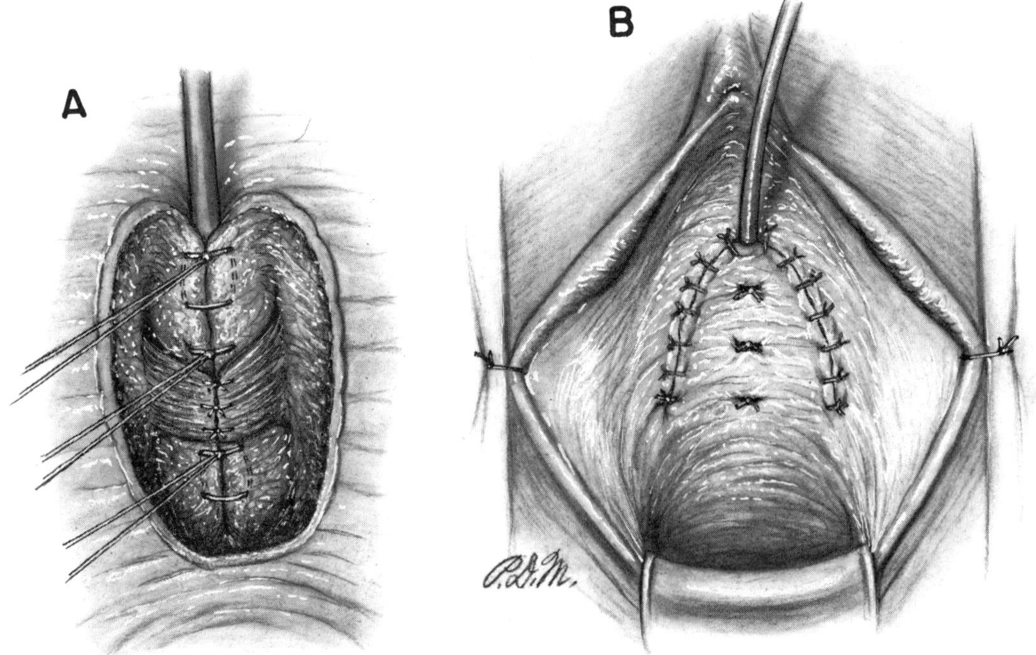

Figure 72.   Reconstruction of the urethra. *A,* A sling of pubococcygeal muscle is used to add support to the vesico-urethral angle. *B,* The previously tied plicating sutures are brought through a mobilized flap of mucosa, and the remaining mucosa is closed with simple sutures.

REVISION OF CONGENITAL MALFORMATIONS

Comments. Gynecologic congenital malformations are many and varied. Because the Lahey Clinic has not been involved in the medical care of infants and young children, only those abnormalities seen in teenagers and young adults and treated by the author will be discussed. Therefore, the mixed external genitalia resulting from hermaphroditism, pseudohermaphroditism, adrenal dysfunction, and hormones will not be considered, except for one patient with mixed genitalia who was seen in her/his late teens. Many patients with testicular feminization and uterine anomalies have been treated via abdominal incisions and will not be discussed. Surgical procedures for congenital malformations are technically far easier than other major abdominal or vaginal operations. Many specialists in gynecologic surgery and general surgeons tend to refer such patients because of a lack of familiarity with the problem rather than a lack of surgical expertise. Although it may be academic to analyze the chromosomes in this group of patients, it is of practical value to confirm the presence of a normal urinary tract by means of preoperative intravenous pyelography. The timing of the operation should be governed by the necessity of the procedure for the patient's health, the ability of the patient to cope with the operation, and the ability and desire of the patient to cooperate in any postoperative program (of particular relevance after construction of a vagina).

Division of Longitudinal Vaginal Septum

Technique. The septum is *divided* and not excised, because an overzealous excision could injure the urethra, bladder, or rectum. After routine preparation and draping of the patient, a No. 14 5 cc Foley catheter is placed into the bladder to permit accurate palpation of the urethra (Fig. 73 *A*). The septum is divided in 1 cm segments from its distal end near the introitus (Fig. 73 *B*). A continuous locking 1–0 chromic catgut suture is begun both anteriorly and posteriorly to close the linear bleeding bed resulting from the incision (Fig. 73 *C*). The 1 cm segments of septum are divided and sutured until the cervix is reached. A double cervix and uterus are usually present, but no attempt is made to divide the cervical septum. The Foley catheter is removed. Gauze impregnated with petroleum jelly is placed in the vagina and removed the next morning before discharge from the hospital.

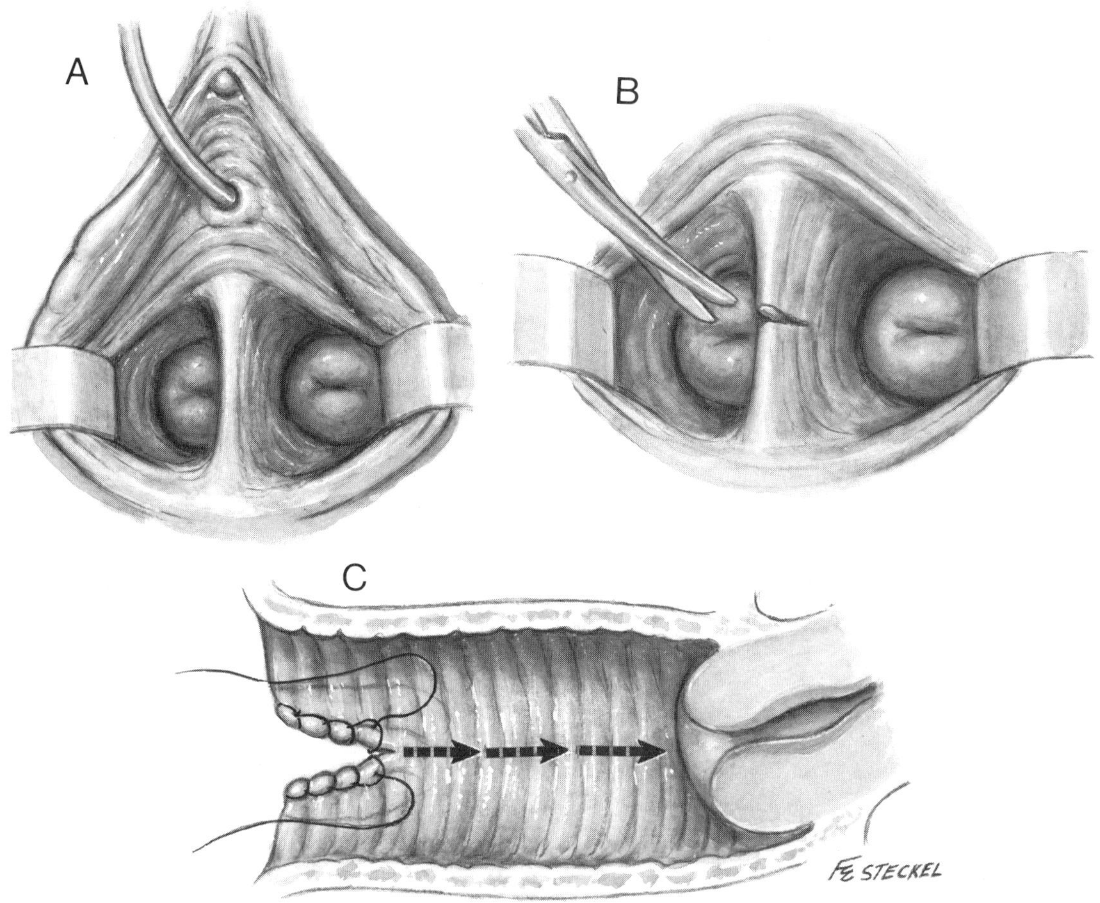

Figure 73.   Division of longitudinal vaginal septum. *A* through *C,* Segmental incision and placement of continuous locking hemostatic sutures.

Division of Transverse Vaginal Septum

Technique.   Occasionally a teenage patient is seen with pelvic discomfort resulting from obstruction of the menstrual flow similar to that seen in a patient with an imperforate hymen but caused by the menstruating uterus being situated above a congenitally absent segment of vagina. In such patients, a bulging upper vagina is located millimeters or centimeters away from a lower vaginal pouch. Examination under anesthesia and with laparoscopy may clarify the extent of the congenital anomaly. After preparation and draping of the patient, a No. 14 5 cc Foley catheter is inserted into the bladder and is left in place to mark the path of the urethra. A small opening is made with a clamp in the exact center of the apex of the vaginal pouch (Fig. 74 *A*). This opening is gently made wider and deeper until the upper segment of vagina is apparent (Fig. 74 *B*). An opening is made into the upper segment with a clamp, resulting in a gush of dark blood. The opening between the upper and lower vagina is gently stretched with the forefinger (Fig. 75 *A*). The lower pouch of the vagina is usually more narrow and may be extended in caliber by a simple vertical incision of the mucosa in the anterior and posterior midlines. The upper and lower segments of the vagina are irrigated thoroughly with saline solution and anastomosed with interrupted 2–0 chromic catgut or polyglycolic acid sutures (Fig. 75 *B*). It is important to hold each suture on tension to provide exposure for placement of the subsequent ones. Prophylactic antibiotic therapy is initiated, a vaginal pack is inserted that extends above the anastomotic site, and the catheter and pack are kept in place until the morning after operation.

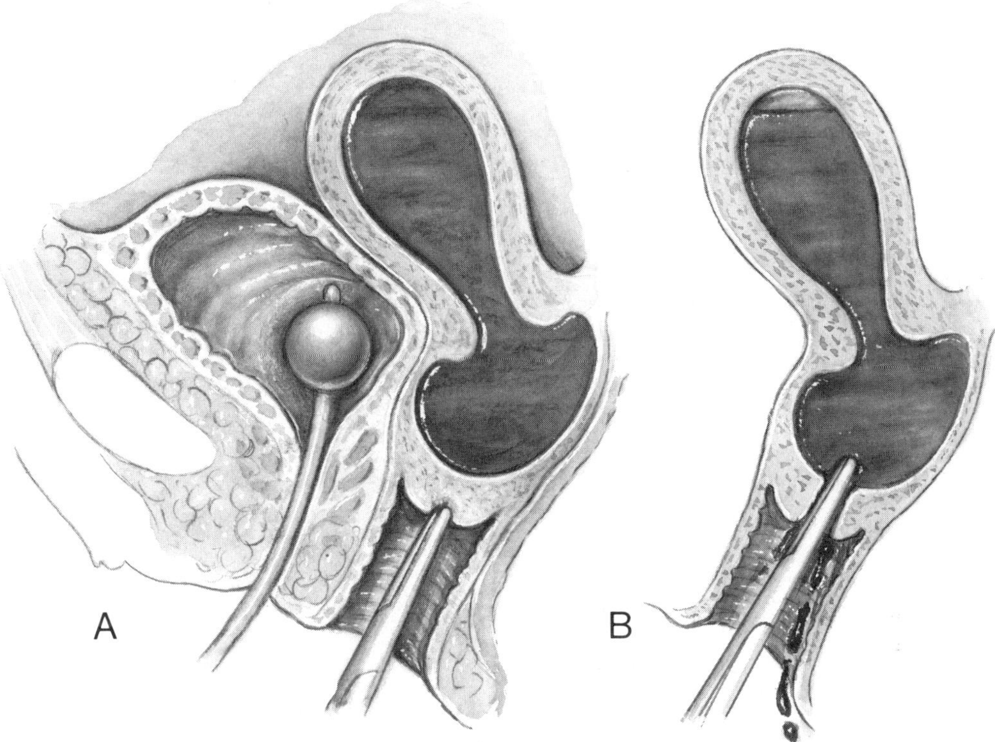

Figure 74. Division of transverse vaginal septum. *A* and *B*, Puncture of septum.

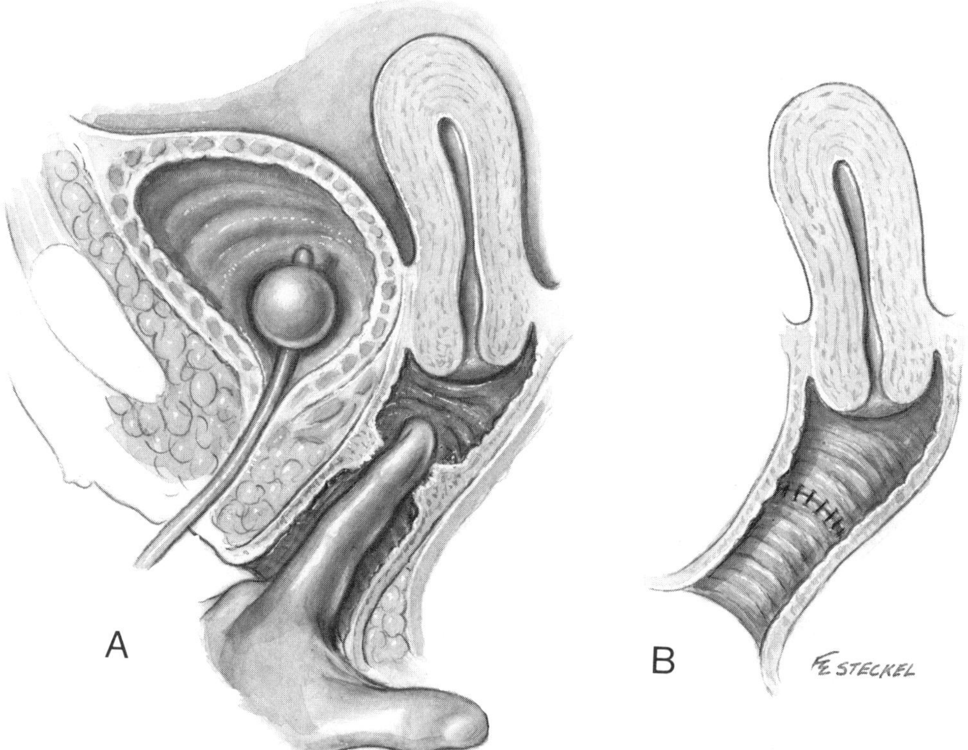

Figure 75. Division of transverse vaginal septum. *A*, Stretching of hole in septum with forefinger. *B*, Anastomosis of upper and lower vagina with simple sutures.

Construction of the Vagina (McIndoe Procedure)

Technique. McIndoe's technique has survived the test of time and represents a quick and easy solution for congenital absence of the vagina. The patient is placed on her side with the top leg flexed at the groin and at the knee, placing the broad surface of the buttocks in view in a somewhat slanted position. The skin of the buttocks is cleaned, shaved, prepared with an antiseptic solution, and draped. The Reese dermatome is set to take the thickest (0.020 inch) split-thickness graft, and the adhesive base is locked into place. Bard-Parker Reese Dermatex compound is placed on the skin of the buttocks with a sterile tongue depressor, allowed to dry momentarily, and the dermatome is pressed firmly against the cemented area of the skin on one end and pulled upward at the same time, while the cutting blade is moved quickly back and forth to produce a uniform graft. The donor graft site is covered with a flat piece of vaginal gauze, which in turn is covered with a loose dressing and held tightly in place with elastic tape. The edges of the skin on the dermatome are grasped with clamps at one edge, and the skin is removed slowly from the adhesive base and placed between two moist sponges.

A catheter is inserted into the bladder, the bladder is emptied, 400 cc of saline are instilled, a quarter-curved Randall kidney stone forceps is inserted through the bladder and through a small suprapubic incision, and a No. 16 Silastic catheter is pulled into the bladder for suprapubic drainage. As with repair of fistulas, in revising congenital anomalies it is wise to have a large-gauge catheter to provide adequate drainage, since the insertion of a catheter through the urethra would be difficult or impossible. At this point a No. 14 5 cc Foley catheter is inserted through the urethra to identify the urethra and bladder during the surgical procedure.

A 1 cm transverse incision is made about 1 cm below the external urethral orifice (Fig. 76 *A*), and this incision is gently increased in depth with a clamp and then with the forefinger (Fig. 76 *B*); *scissors should never be used.* When the urethra is used as a guide, the potential vaginal space is easily opened. The middle region of the vaginal space tends to be somewhat constricted, and some surgeons prefer to divide this area of thickening, but it is not necessary in most instances. Active focal bleeding is controlled with superficial 3–0 chromic catgut sutures; oozing is controlled by the insertion of a moist vaginal pack or sponge.

For many years a variety of sterile balsa wood molds have been available to be fashioned to the individual needs of each patient. These molds are covered with two condoms and anchored with heavy silk to a metal eye screw inserted into the flat end of the mold. However, recently we have changed to the large polyethylene mold used by Evans of Detroit.* This well-designed mold simplifies the procedure. The skin from the site of the donor graft is placed on the mold, and its edges are approximated with 4–0 chromic catgut so that the skin covers the entire mold evenly (Fig. 76 *C*).

The moistened pack is removed from the vaginal space, the mold is put into place, and its edges are sutured to the mucosa of the introitus (Fig. 77 *A*). The labia majora are then closed over the introitus with simple interrupted No. 2 Tevdek sutures (Fig. 77 *B*). Prophylactic antibiotics are begun in the operating room and continued for five days. One week after operation the patient returns to the operating room, is lightly anesthetized, and the dressing is changed over the donor graft site on the buttocks, the labial sutures are removed, the mold is removed, and the newly created vagina is irrigated with saline. If the same mold can fit snugly in the vagina and be retained naturally, it is used. If not, a new mold is fashioned with small cubes of foam rubber placed within two condoms. The patient is discharged the next morning with the indwelling mold and suprapubic catheter still in place, and she returns to the office in two weeks.

---

*Obtainable from the Troy Scientific Corporation, 1023 Troy Court, Troy, Michigan 48084.

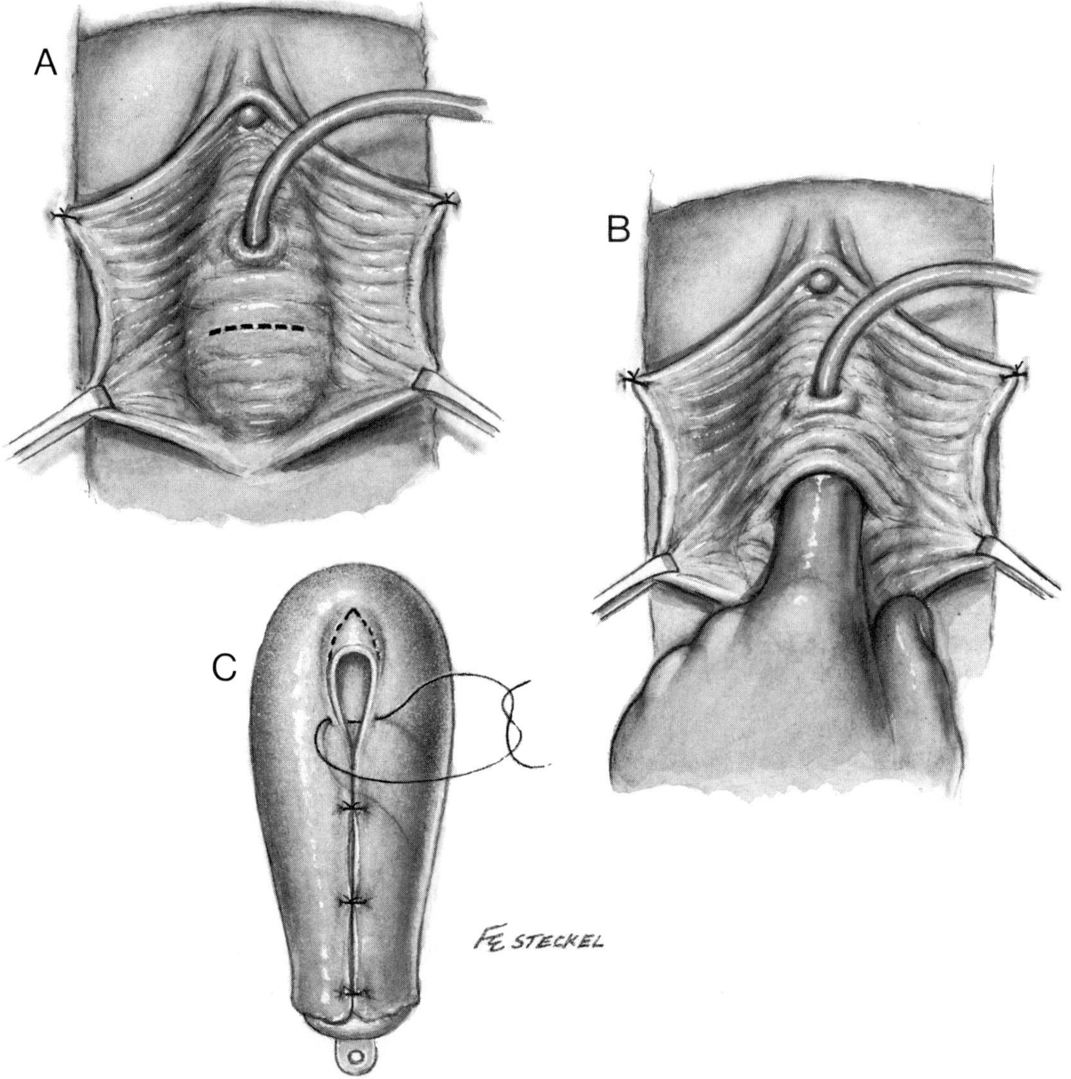

Figure 76.　Construction of vagina (McIndoe procedure). *A,* A 1 cm transverse incision (dashed line) is made about 1 cm below the external urethral orifice. *B,* The space between the urethra and bladder and rectum is gently developed with a forefinger. *C,* Placement of split-thickness skin graft over a polyethylene mold to form a perfect fit.

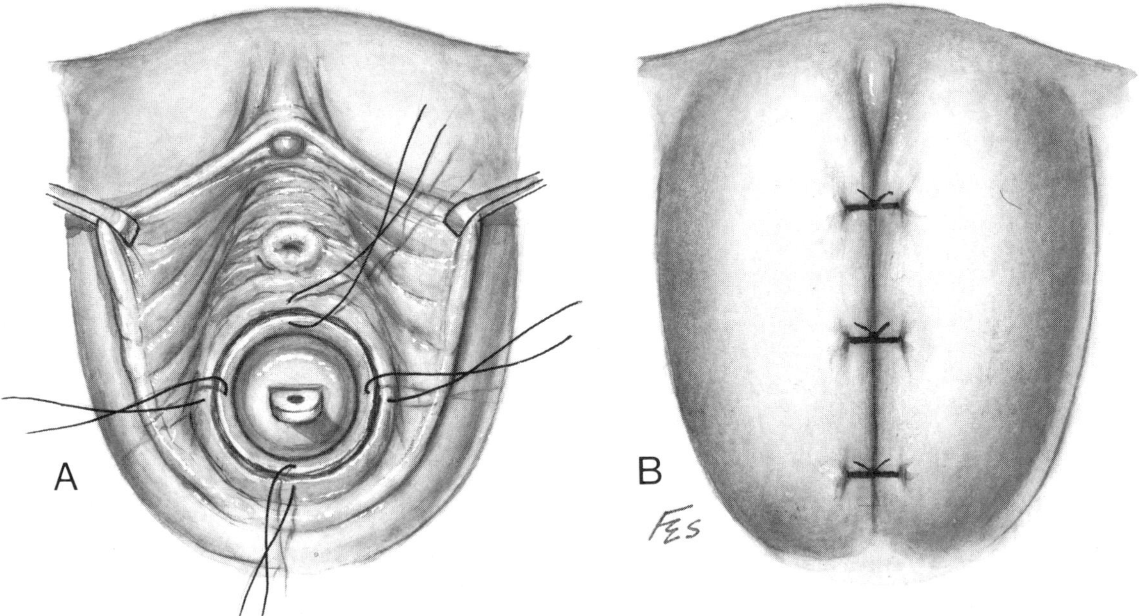

Figure 77.   Construction of vagina (McIndoe procedure). *A,* The skin-covered mold is placed into the vaginal space and its edges sutured to the mucosa around the introitus. *B,* The labia majora are approximated with heavy Tevdek sutures.

Construction of Vagina and Uterovaginal Canal

Comments.   Only a few cases have been reported in the medical literature of patients requiring construction of both a vagina and uterovaginal canal, for the congenital absence of both cervix and vagina is rare indeed. The history of the one patient in my experience is presented and the technique is described.

Technique.   A 14-year-old patient was transferred to our gynecology service after exploratory laparotomy for an acute abdomen had revealed blood flowing back through the tubes from a large, bulging bicornuate uterus; the surgeon had been aware of the absence of the vagina. An opening had been made into the uterus, and the surgeon could neither palpate nor visualize a cervix, and he had been unable to detect or probe a cervical canal from within the uterine cavity. A mushroom catheter had been placed through the abdominal wall into the uterine cavity for drainage, and the abdomen had been closed. At this point, in order to gain time before further surgical intervention,

menstruation was stopped and suppressed with oral contraceptives. Antibiotics were continued until the catheter was removed and the patient became afebrile.

Three months after laparotomy, a combined abdominovaginal approach was made to correct the anomaly. A routine McIndoe construction of the vagina was begun. A split-thickness segment of skin was placed directly over a balsa wood mold in which a 0.25 inch (0.635 cm) hole had been drilled through its vertical center. The vaginal space was packed with moist gauze and a Foley catheter left in place in the bladder. The abdomen had been prepared and draped in continuity with the genital area. Laparotomy was performed. Since an incision had to be made into the uterus, the septum of the bicornuate uterus was incised. A long Kelly clamp was used to make a connection between the uterine cavity and the newly created vaginal space. Two plastic tubes were placed down through the uterine cavity, through the newly created canal between the uterus and the vagina, and through the opening in the vaginal mold as the mold (covered with the skin graft) was inserted into the vaginal space as for routine construction of the vagina (Fig. 78). The abdominal sides of the tubes were brought out through separate openings in the uterus and abdominal wall, sealed with heat, and tied over the abdomen to prevent slippage. The lower portions of the tubes were also sealed and tied just below the vaginal mold. The skin of the graft was anchored to the introitus, and the vulva was closed over the introitus with No. 2 Tevdek sutures. The uterus was closed, thereby unifying the uterine cavity. The bladder was distended with saline solution, and a suprapubic Foley catheter was inserted into the bladder. The abdominal wall was closed in routine fashion. Prophylactic antibiotics were given, and suppression of menstruation with hormones was continued.

Sixteen days after operation, the dressing over the donor graft site was changed, the vaginal mold was removed, and the plastic tubes were shortened to the abdominal wall and to the opening to the uterus and anchored in place with polyethylene buttons. A new mold, without a center hole, was fashioned for the vagina and put into place. The patient was discharged from the hospital on the following day.

One month after the reconstruction operation, the plastic tubes were removed via the vagina, and a Silastic shield was put into the uterine cavity with its string going through a large plastic tube used to splint the newly constructed canal between the uterine cavity and vagina. Six months after the reconstruction operation, oral contraceptive treatment was stopped, and the patient resumed her menses via the vagina. A wax mold was inserted only at night. Six weeks after stopping the oral contraceptives, the plastic splint was removed, but the shield within the uterine cavity was left in place.

The string receded out of sight, and the shield was left in place in the uterine cavity rather than impose further trauma on the patient. The Silastic shield was removed with the patient under anesthesia in January 1977, five and a half years after the original reconstruction operation.

Remarks. Upon review of the technique employed here and elsewhere for this rare anomaly, a different approach is proposed for the future — performing this procedure in two stages, after clarification of the diagnosis through examination under anesthesia and with laparoscopy, if required. If menses have begun or begin before the completion of the procedure, it is wise to suppress menstruation with hormones. The first stage would be routine vaginal construction. The second stage would be four months later, when a laparotomy would be performed, and the uterine cavity would be exposed through a short anterior midline incision in the uterine fundus. A long Kelly clamp would be used to connect the uterine cavity with the vagina, and a large Silastic tube would be tied in a loop within the uterine cavity and the vaginal end of the tube anchored to the upper vagina with a polyethylene button. Menstruation would be suppressed for three more months, at which time the patient could menstruate. The Silastic splint would be removed, preferably after regular menses had been established. Such a two-stage procedure would simplify the treatment of this rare congenital anomaly.

A variation of this basic technical concept has been reported by Farber and Marchant (1976) with good results. A dissenting viewpoint has been presented by Maciulla and associates (1978) and by Niver et al. (1980), who believe that the uterine fundus should be removed.

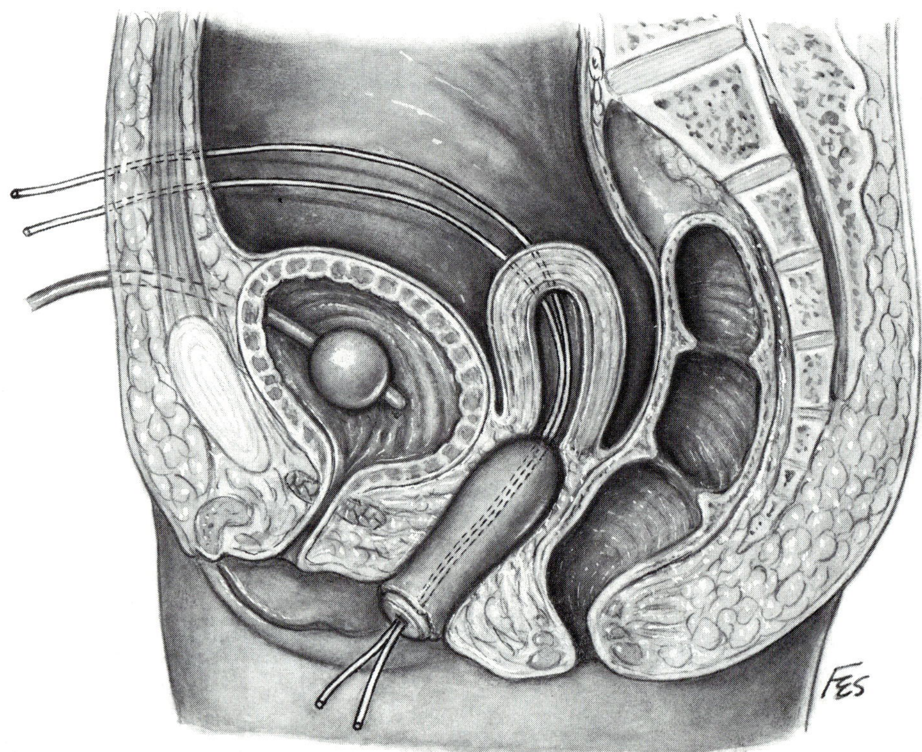

Figure 78.   Construction of vagina and uterovaginal canal. Plastic tubes are placed through the uterine cavity, through an artificial opening to a newly created vaginal space, and through a central canal of the skin-covered vaginal mold.

Construction of Genital Pouch (Modified Williams Procedure)

Comments. This modification of the Williams procedure is perhaps the simplest procedure to create a pouch that can function as a vagina. It produces the same septum that would be divided in infancy when associated with female pseudohermaphroditism, the adrenogenital syndrome, or intrauterine virilization secondary to hormone therapy. The procedure may be employed not only for congenital absence of the vagina but also for other instances of vaginal stenosis and shortening.

Technique. A wide, large U-shaped incision is made just inside the labia majora, with the top points of the U at the level of the urethral orifice and the base of the U at the lowest point on the vulva (Fig. 79 *A*). The caliber of the new vagina will be about one third the width of the U. The medial edge of the U is mobilized at its base to permit approximation with interrupted 2–0 chromic catgut sutures (Fig. 79 *B*). A final or second layer of 2–0 Tevdek sutures is used to approximate the outer edge of the U (Fig. 79 *C*). Prophylactic antibiotics are begun. The No. 12 Cystocath suprapubic catheter is left in place when the patient is discharged on the fourth postoperative day. The patient returns for removal of the Tevdek sutures and catheter two weeks later. At one month after the operation the patient is instructed to initiate dilatation of the pouch and formation of a vagina, starting with insertion of a wax candle or dilator 2 cm in diameter.

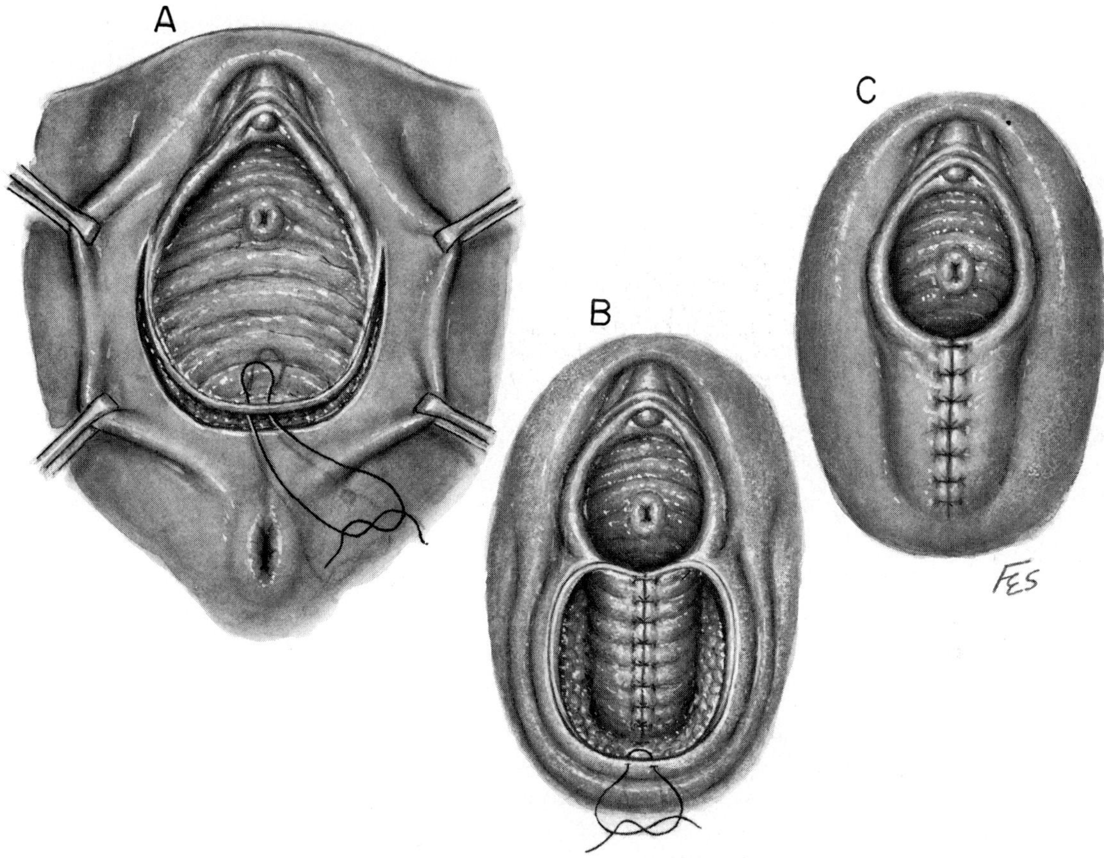

Figure 79. Construction of genital pouch (modified Williams procedure). *A*, A wide, **U**-shaped incision is made with the top points at the level of the urethral orifice, the arms just inside the labia majora, and the base at the fourchette. *B*, The incision is deepened, the tissue mobilized, and the medial flap approximated with simple catgut sutures. *C*, The outer or final layer is closed with deep Tevdek sutures.

Restoration of Normal Position of the Vagina and the Vulva After Exstrophy of the Bladder

Comments. In the future more patients with exstrophy of the bladder will survive to adulthood with functioning ileal bladders. In such patients the pubic rami are separated, and the labia majora diverge toward the lower part of the abdomen above the groin, with the vaginal introitus often narrowed and displaced superiorly.

Technique. The lower abdomen and genital area are prepared and draped, and the ileal bladder is covered with a plastic drape to prevent contamination. A vertical incision is made below the vaginal introitus to the point of desired transplantation in the perineal area (Fig. 80). The vaginal opening is circumscribed with an incision (Fig. 80), and the lower vagina is mobilized, brought down to its new site, and sutured in place with 2–0 Tevdek sutures (Fig. 81). The vaginal introitus may be narrow so that short vertical mucosal incisions may be necessary to increase its caliber before it is sutured to the skin in its new location. The skin tends to be rigid in this area. An inverted V-shaped incision is made over the divergent labium majus on each side, and the labia with adjacent fat are mobilized medially and approximated with No. 1 and 2–0 Tevdek sutures above the transplanted vaginal introitus, simulating the normal genital anatomy (Fig. 82). Do *not* extend the midline incision upward from the original location of the vaginal opening, for the abdominal wall may be quite thin at this point after previous cystectomy. The skin defects resulting from mobilization of the flaps of the vulva may be closed with No. 1 Tevdek sutures; the skin and fat may require mobilization to permit approximation. Prophylactic antibiotics are begun during operation. A tight dressing is applied. The patient should remain in the hospital for one week and return for removal of sutures three weeks after operation.

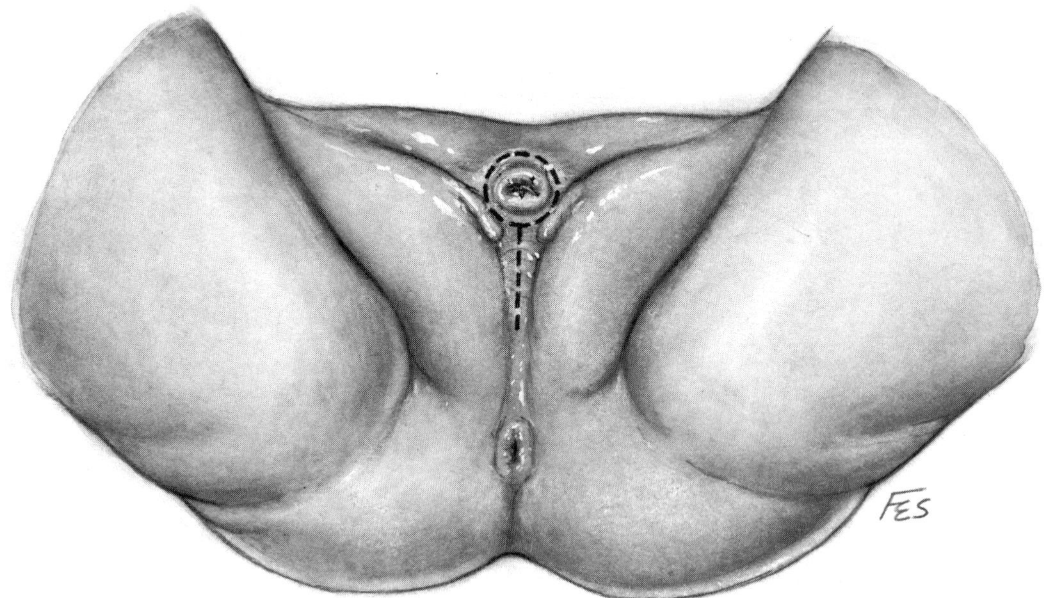

Figure 80. Restoration of normal position of vagina and vulva after exstrophy of the bladder. The initial incision circumscribes the displaced vaginal introitus and extends below it in the vertical midline to a point 2 cm above the anal margin.

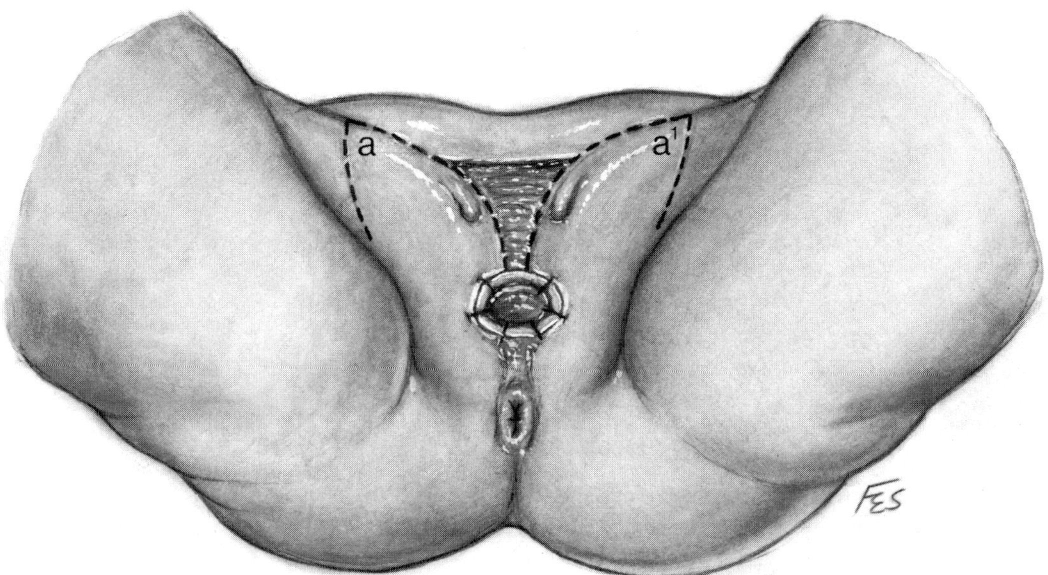

Figure 81.   Restoration of normal position of vagina and vulva after exstrophy of the bladder. The distal vagina is mobilized and brought down to its new site. The dashed lines show the incisions for mobilization of the divergent labia majora (a and a¹).

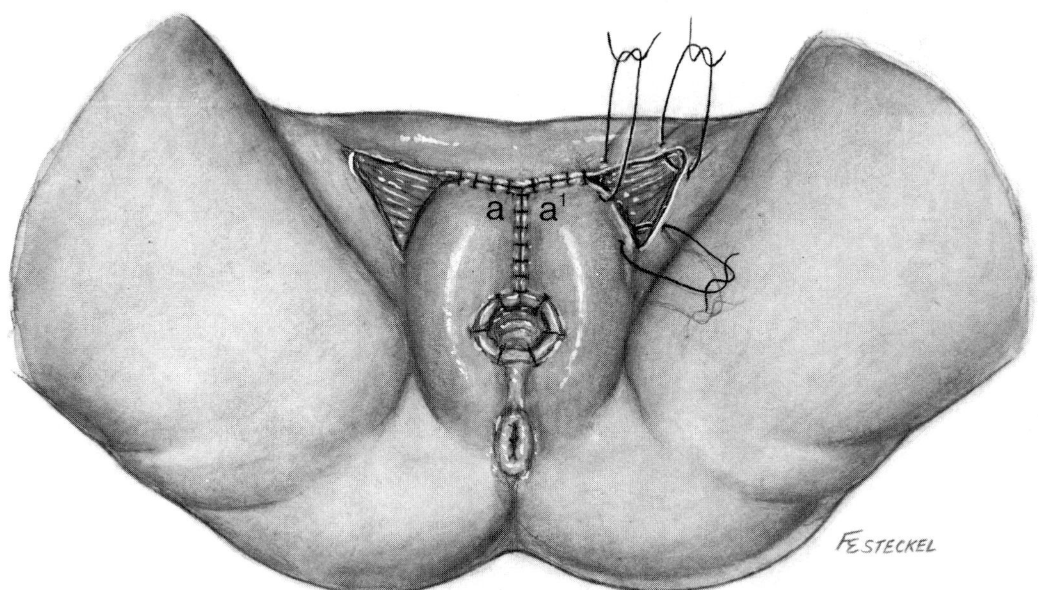

Figure 82.   Restoration of normal position of vagina and vulva after exstrophy of the bladder. The upper divergent vulva (a and a¹) is mobilized and transplanted to a position above the vaginal introitus.

Excision of Testes and Phallus Remnant

Comments. The young adult patient with mixed genitalia whom we treated had a normal male chromosomal analysis, testes within the inguinal canal, male breasts, and mixed external genitalia consisting of a 4 cm phallus, a urethral orifice beneath the phallus, a 2 cm vaginal pouch, and a fatty fold on each side of the pouch resembling a vulva more than a scrotal sac. Gender identification at birth and since was as a female.

Technique. A low transverse abdominal incision was made, the inguinal canals opened, and the testes removed with ease. The inguinal canals were closed to prevent future hernias. The phallus was circumscribed around its upper half by a superficial incision while preserving a segment of skin on its undersurface (Fig. 83), and the phallus was excised as close as possible to its origin beneath the symphysis pubis. After closure of the operative defect with a vertical line of 2–0 chromic catgut sutures, the segment of preserved skin simulated the clitoris (Fig. 84). An alternative with a small phallus is to remove its anterior half, reserving the glans and corpora cavernosa to simulate the clitoris. A small vertical incision was made at the posterior midline of the vaginal pouch, and this incision was closed transversely with simple sutures (Fig. 85). The patient has been receiving estrogen therapy for many years with fair breast development, but she has not desired creation of a functional vagina by means of dilators or operation.

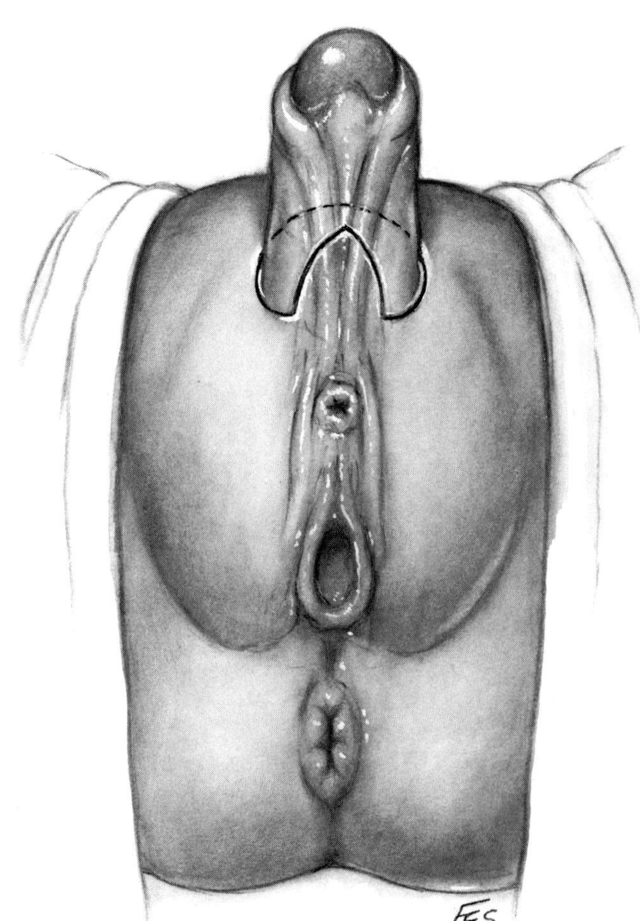

Figure 83. Excision of phallus remnant. A circumscribing incision is made around the upper half of the base of the phallus, and an elliptical segment of skin is preserved on the undersurface of the phallus.

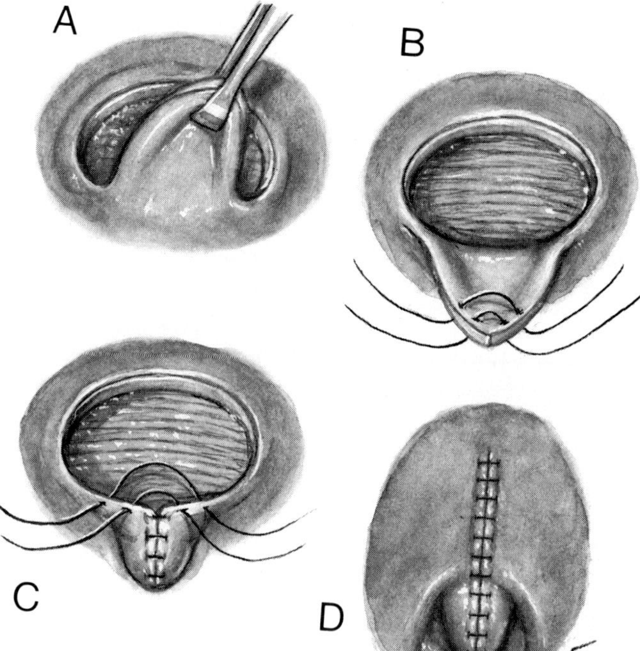

Figure 84. Excision of phallus remnant. *A* through *D,* The inner surface of the preserved segment of skin is closed with simple sutures to create a tag of skin simulating the clitoris. The remaining operative defect is closed with simple sutures.

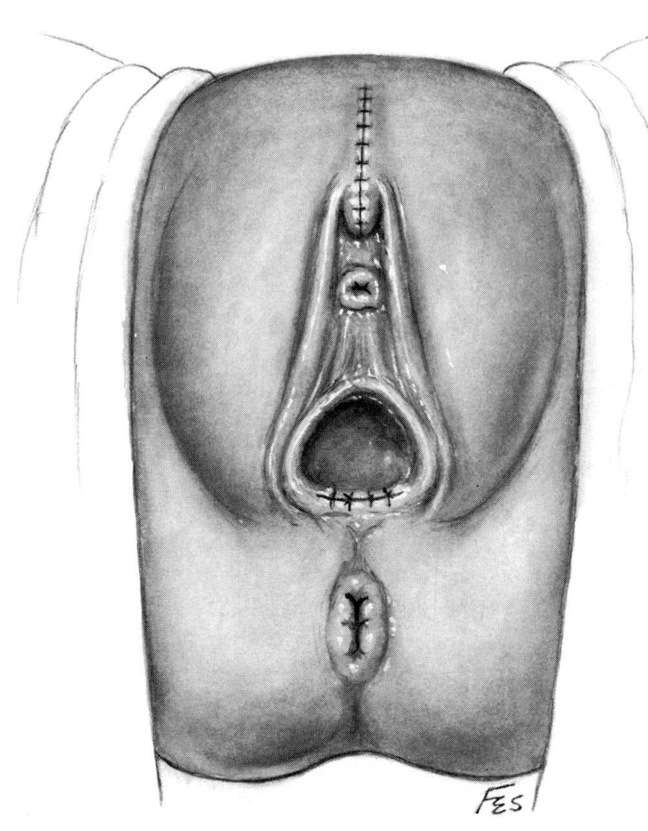

Figure 85. Excision of phallus remnant. The posterior vaginal outlet has been revised with a short vertical midline incision, followed by transverse closure with simple sutures.

Overall Postoperative Considerations

Correction of a longitudinal or transverse septum of the vagina involves minimal trauma to tissue so that the patient may be up and about quickly. Division of the transverse septum does involve release of old blood, which may have caused distention and edema of the upper vaginal pouch; therefore prophylactic antibiotics are employed in such situations. An indwelling catheter is not used.

Any construction of the vagina, except the Williams procedure, requires an indwelling suprapubic bladder catheter of larger caliber than the Cystocath. Such suprapubic bladder drainage has virtually eliminated necrosis of the urethra and also eliminates use of a foreign body in the vaginal operative site. Whether the mold is made of balsa wood, plastic material, or foam rubber, it is paramount that it remain in place for one month and that it be inserted into the vagina every night until frequent coitus occurs. In my experience, the one failure, which required revision of vaginal stenosis, resulted from either the patient's lack of understanding of maintaining the mold or the surgeon's inability to convey the importance of this point. If a plastic mold fits perfectly and can be retained by the tone of the introitus, this is the first choice. Otherwise, balsa wood covered with a condom, foam rubber cubes covered with a condom, or an oval wax candle may be used. All of these methods permit the surgeon to fashion the device to the needs of the patient.

The construction of a uterovaginal canal with creation of the vagina requires special emphasis on maintaining the canal until smooth epithelium lines the entire surface of the canal. Suppression of menses combined with a large Silastic tubular splint serves this purpose.

The Williams procedure requires only a suprapubic catheter (No. 12 Cystocath) so that the patient does not void for two weeks.

After surgical correction of the genital anomaly associated with exstrophy of the bladder, it is wise to keep the Tevdek sutures in place for three weeks, for there is tension at the donor site of the vulva skin flaps, and the skin is usually tense as a result of previous surgery for the exposed bladder.

Care after revision of mixed external genitalia must be individualized, but, for the case presented, the patient was only limited by an indwelling Foley catheter for 48 hours and resumed normal diet and ambulation the day after operation. The hospital stay was limited to one week.

DENERVATION OF VULVA (MERING PROCEDURE)

Comments. Denervation of the vulva is a rare procedure and should be employed when pruritus vulvae is unresponsive to conservative management and in the absence of any vulvar and vaginal disease. Its use should be limited to resolving pruritus only and should not be applied to the relief of pain.

Technique. The lower part of the abdomen and genitoanal area are prepared and draped. A 2 cm vertical incision is made **between** the labium minus and labium majus on each side, extending to the fascia. The surgeon's forefinger is used to undermine the vulvar and perianal areas (Fig. 86). A Hemovac drain is placed through a separate puncture site on each side at the base of the vulva. The incisions are closed with simple 2–0 Tevdek sutures. A suprapubic No. 12 Cystocath is inserted. The operative site is covered with a tight dressing. This is the most important step in preventing postoperative hematoma and infection. Prophylactic antibiotics are begun at the time of operation.

Postoperative Considerations. Intravenous fluids are continued for three days.

On the third postoperative day the suction tubes are removed if drainage is minimal. On the fourth postoperative day the dressing is removed, and the patient is allowed to void and to resume a regular diet. The supra- pubic catheter is removed when the patient is able to void normally, and discharge is planned for the fifth postoperative day after removal of the sutures.

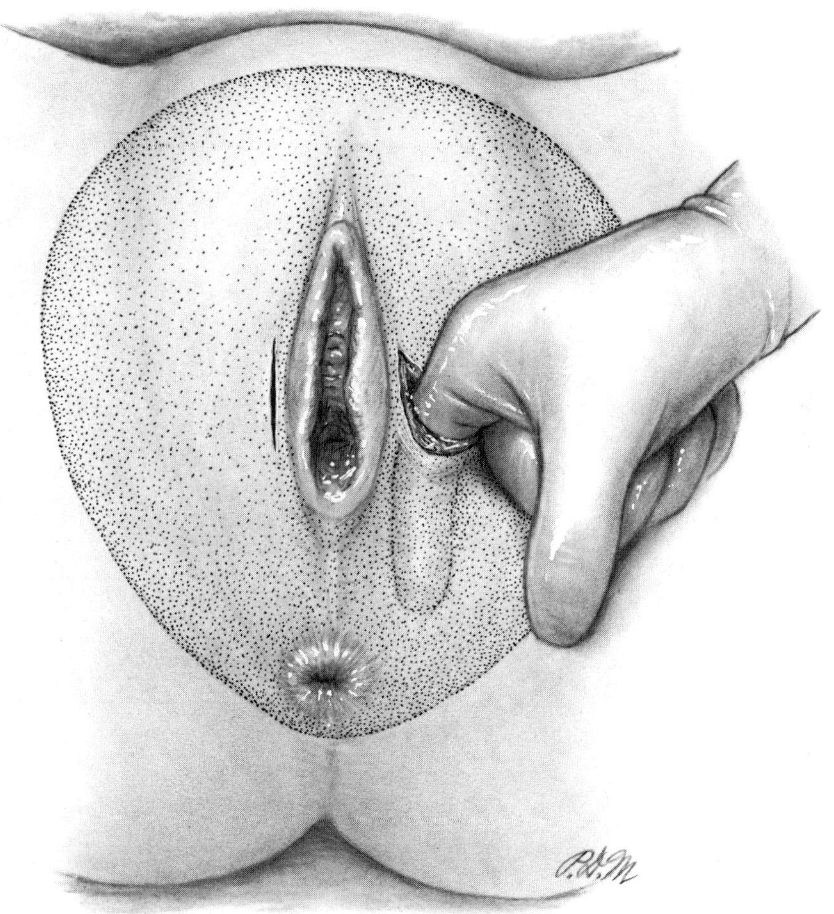

Figure 86. Denervation of vulva (modified Mering procedure). Short vertical incisions are made in the fold between the labia majora and labia minora. The finger is used to mobilize the skin and adjacent fat over a wide area involved by intractable pruritus.

REVISION OF NARROWED INTROITUS

Comments. The natural narrowing of the introitus by the hymen is discussed under the section on minor surgery. Also, a natural narrowing may occur with exstrophy of the bladder and with the anomalous existence of a flap of skin covering the introitus and urethra (see Williams procedure), as discussed elsewhere. Beyond these instances, the need for revision of the introitus should be rare in the young woman. Appropriate reassurance, trial of coitus, and vaginal dilators (a set of four Young's dilators) should be employed.

Perineorrhaphy and vulvectomy are the commonest causes of narrowed introitus. Many such strictures may be prevented at the time of initial operation, but the perfect operative result at age 35 may be transformed by aging and diminished coitus to functional narrowing of the vaginal introitus at age 55. The raised or "dashboard" perineum secondary to operation can be corrected by simple perineal revision. Uniform stricture of the introitus may be managed best by the Z-plasty.

Rarely a patient may be seen who has a snug introitus, a low urethral orifice, and recurrent cystitis and urethritis after coitus. When other causes of infection have been ruled out, simple revision of the anterior introitus may be performed to displace the external urethral orifice anteriorly. This procedure is not employed in the presence of dyspareunia; in such a patient perineal revision or Z-plasty is best.

Simple Revision of Perineum

Technique. After routine genital preparation and draping, a vertical incision is made for 2 to 3 cm at the posterior midline of the introitus (Fig. 87 *A*). The vaginal mucosa is undermined and mobilized with Metzenbaum scissors (Fig. 87 *B*), and the incision is closed in a transverse direction with simple 2–0 Tevdek sutures (Fig. 87 *C*). An indwelling catheter is not used, and the patient is discharged the following day and returns for suture removal in 10 days.

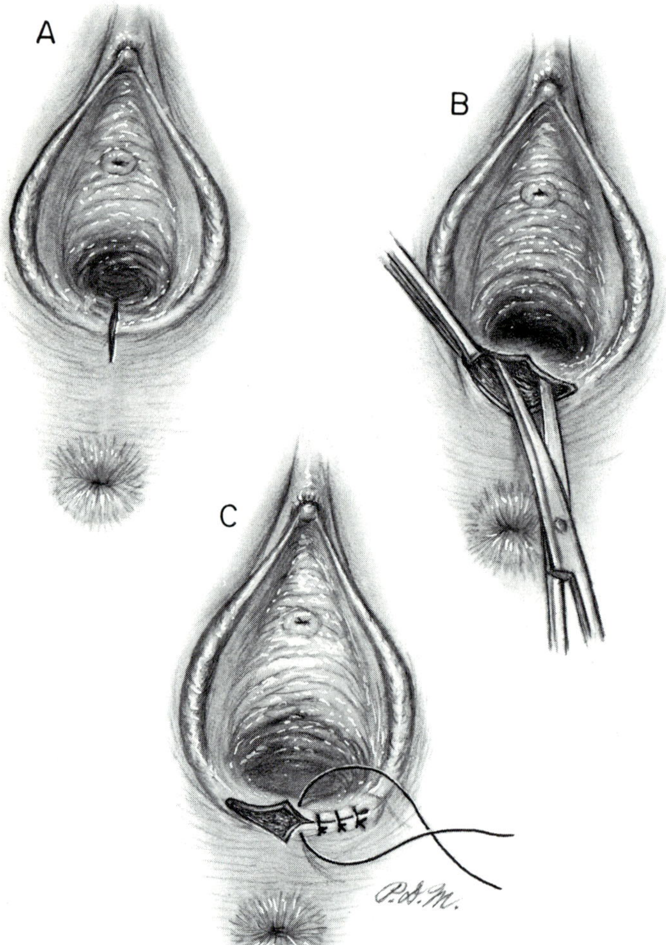

Figure 87. Simple perineal revision of stenosed introitus. *A,* A short vertical incision at the perineal and introital midline. *B,* Mobilization of the mucosa. *C,* Transverse closure with simple sutures.

Z-plasty

Technique. The lower abdomen and genital area are prepared and draped. A Z-shaped incision is made on each side of the introitus (Fig. 88 *A*) down to include the subcutaneous fat, and flaps are mobilized and transposed (Fig. 88 *B*), thereby increasing the lateral rim of the introitus by 1 cm or more. The skin is approximated with simple 2–0 Tevdek sutures (Fig. 88 *C*). A No. 12 Cystocath is inserted into the bladder and removed before the patient is discharged from the hospital on the third postoperative day. A tight dressing is applied at the end of the operation and kept in place for two days, at which time the patient is allowed to void. Sutures are removed on or around the 10th postoperative day.

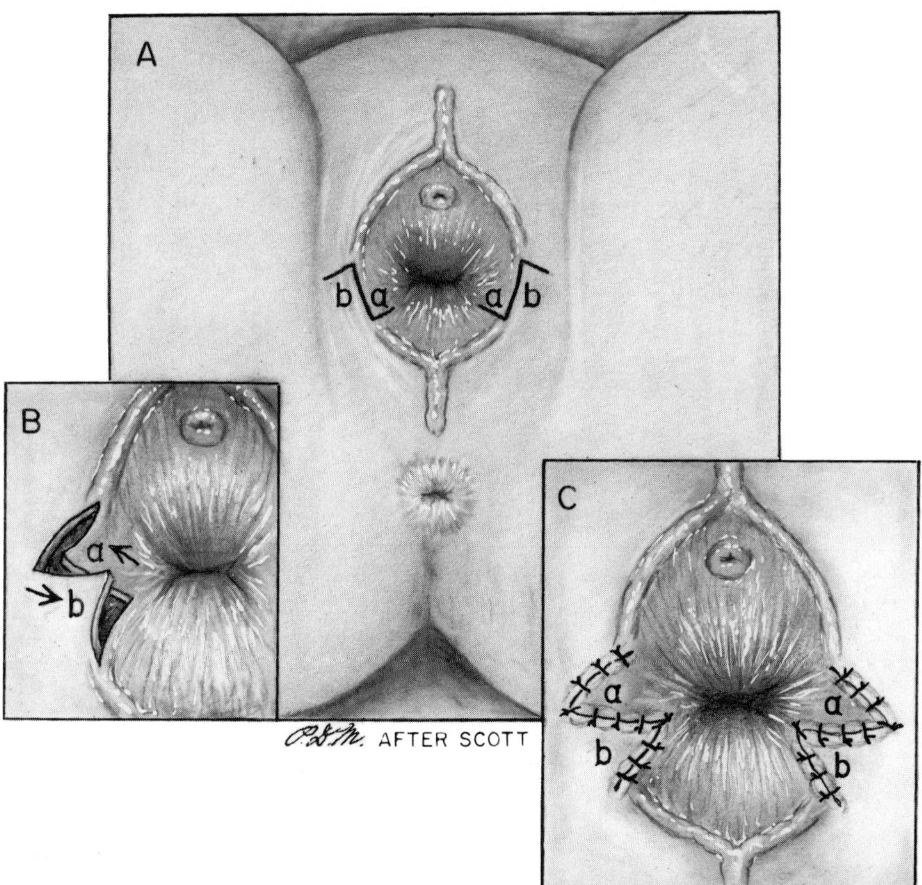

Figure 88. **Z**-plasty for stenosed introitus. *A*, **Z** incisions at lateral margins of constricted introitus. *B*, Triangular flaps of mucosa and skin are mobilized and reversed. *C*, Final closure with simple sutures.

Elevation of Urethral Orifice

Technique. This procedure simply raises the urethral orifice to a position away from a snug introitus and away from the direct trauma produced by coitus. In contrast to the former two procedures, it is not used for dyspareunia and does not increase the size of the introitus. After routine preparation and draping of the genital area, a 1 cm transverse incision is made about 3 mm below the urethral orifice (Fig. 89 *A*). This incision is then closed vertically with 3–0 chromic catgut sutures (Fig. 89 *B* and *C*). A catheter is not used, a dressing is not applied, and the patient is discharged on the morning after operation.

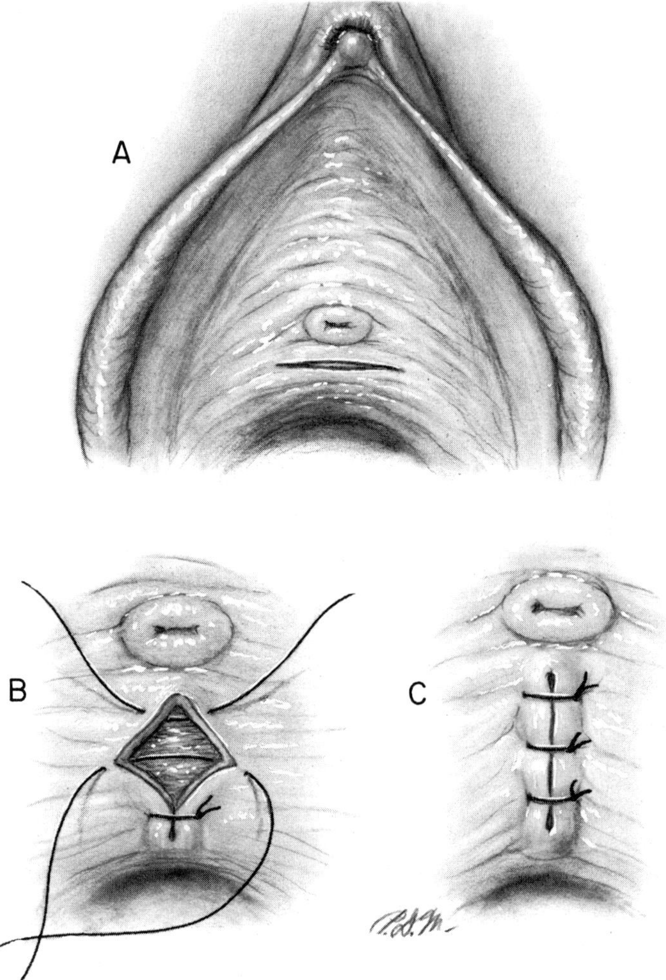

Figure 89.   Elevation of urethral orifice. *A,* Transverse mucosal incision 1 cm long and 0.3 cm below urethral orifice. *B* and *C,* Vertical closure with simple sutures.

Overall Postoperative Considerations

Perineal revision and revision of the urethral orifice impose minimal trauma and are managed as minor procedures except for the delay in removal of the sutures for the perineal operation. The added trauma of the Z-plasty has been managed conservatively with the suprapubic catheter, the use of nonabsorbing sutures, and a five-day hospitalization. When the mucosa is atrophic and rigid in association with the postmenopausal state, it may be prudent to prescribe conjugated estrogens, 0.3 mg daily for the first 25 days of the month, or to prescribe an intravaginal estrogen cream daily (one half an applicator) for two weeks, followed by a maintenance dose twice weekly.

VULVECTOMY

Simple Vulvectomy

Comments. During the past two decades a welcome trend toward conservatism has appeared regarding the use of simple vulvectomy. Simple vulvectomy for leukoplakia, intractable vulvitis, and intractable pruritus vulvae is no longer justified. Indeed, does any indication exist for simple vulvectomy? Perhaps it is warranted in the presence of *bilateral, multifocal,* severe dysplasia of the vulva; carcinoma in situ of the vulva; and *superficial* Paget's disease. Otherwise, when the disease is localized, wide excision of the lesion would be more appropriate than simple vulvectomy.

Technique. The lower abdomen and genital area are prepared and draped. A superficial incision is made around the introitus extending 1 cm above the external urethral orifice. A similar incision outlines the outer margin of the vulvectomy, making certain that a margin of 1 cm of normal skin is excised beyond the lesions. Similarly, the depth of the vulvectomy should be sufficient to permit adequate examination of tissue by the pathologist — approximately 1 cm. Excision is begun at the upper margin of the outer incision. The tissue to be removed is placed on tension, and the skin and subcutaneous fat are simply excised with the scalpel. Many small bleeding blood vessels are encountered, clamped, and ligated; a figure-of-eight suture is placed around the clitoris proximal to the site of excision. The surgeon must glance back and forth at the urethral orifice to assess the location of the urethra. A Kelly clamp pushed upward from the inner incision helps to identify the anterior borders of the specimen to be removed (Fig. 90). The lateral aspect of the vulvectomy is performed with ease by connecting the inner and outer incisions with the excision of an appropriate depth of subcutaneous fat. With excision of the posterior portion of the vulva and perineum, care must be taken to avoid injury to the anus and rectum. At this point it is wise to dissect downward from the posterior vaginal introitus toward the outer incision of the perineum. After the specimen has been removed and hemostasis obtained, the posterior vaginal mucosa is mobilized and the underlying levators are plicated, if necessary. Subcutaneous sutures are no longer used in the closure, but simple No. 1 Tevdek sutures are used to approximate tissue under tension and 2–0 Tevdek sutures to approximate mucosa and skin with minimal tension (Fig. 91). Simple vertical approximation of the skin to cover the upper defect will reduce the tension between the mucosa of the skin on the upper and lateral borders of the introitus (Fig. 92). For simple vulvectomy, no drains are used. A No. 12 suprapubic Cystocath catheter is placed in the bladder, and a tight dressing is applied.

Postoperative Considerations. Prophylactic antibiotics are not given routinely. Intravenous fluids are continued until the fourth postoperative day, when the dressing is removed and the patient is permitted to ambulate. The patient is permitted to void on the sixth postoperative day, and the suprapubic catheter may be removed on the following morning. Discharge from the hospital is planned for the eighth postoperative day, and the patient returns to the office two weeks after discharge for removal of the sutures. It is important for the patient to receive perineal care twice daily and after bowel movements in the hospital (after the removal of the dressing) and to take a brief warm bath after each bowel movement at home to reduce contamination of the operative site.

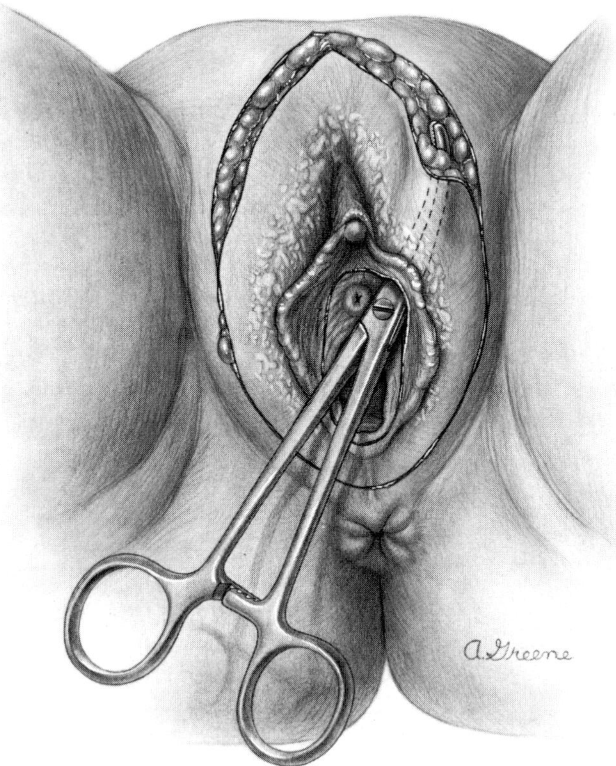

Figure 90. Simple vulvectomy. Incisions outline borders of vulvectomy, and a clamp undermines depth of tissue to be removed.

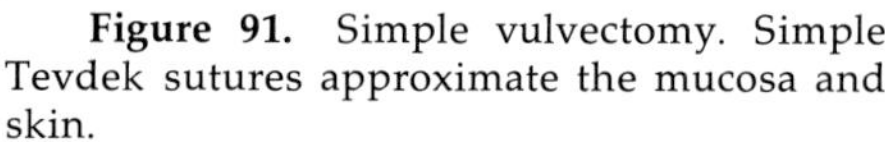

Figure 91. Simple vulvectomy. Simple Tevdek sutures approximate the mucosa and skin.

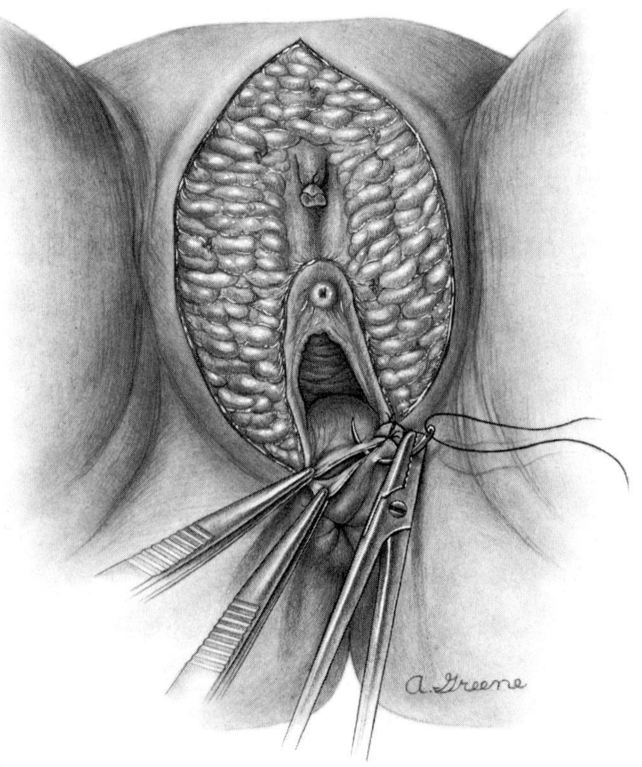

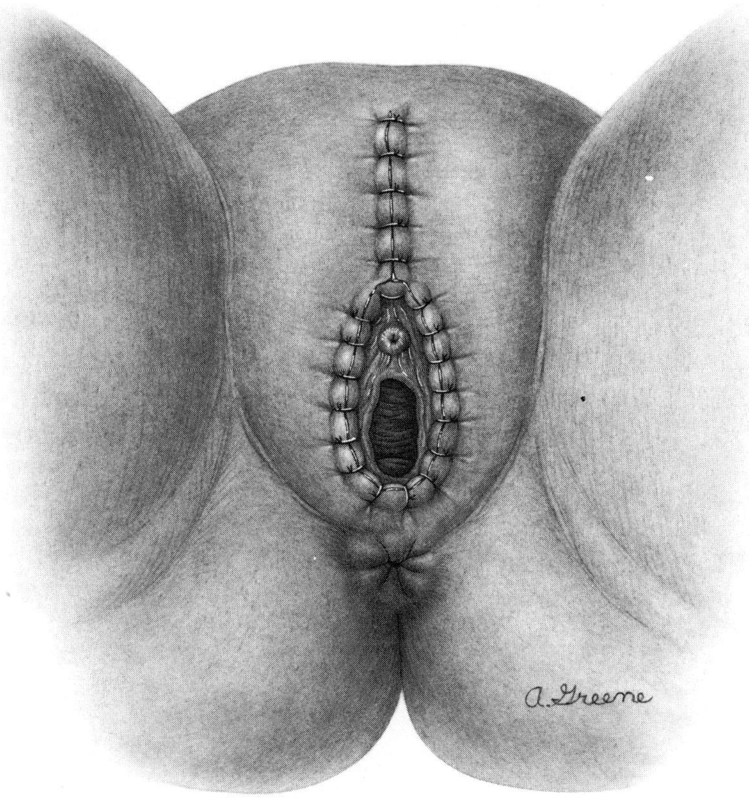

Figure 92. Simple vulvectomy. Simple vertical approximation of the upper defect will reduce the tension between the upper and lateral borders of the mucosa and skin.

Radical Vulvectomy

Comments. Radical vulvectomy without lymphadenectomy represents a compromise in the optimal treatment of squamous cell carcinoma of the vulva. This method is selected either in an effort to reduce the trauma and risk of surgery for the poor-risk patient or in the hope that a surgical cure may be achieved for a small, localized, and well-differentiated carcinoma. In the former instance supplementary irradiation may be directed to the groin and pelvic nodes. In the latter instance the logic of radical vulvectomy may be questioned, since a wide, deep excision of the tumor should provide a cure if the carcinoma is localized. The treatment of vulvar carcinoma will be explored further in the next section.

Technique. The lower part of the abdomen and genital area are prepared and draped. As in the simple vulvectomy, the extent of operation is outlined by inner and outer incisions. The operation proceeds in the same way as the simple procedure except that the dissection extends deep to the fascia, dipping in below the pubic rami before the clitoris is excised, and requires more care to avoid injury to the urethra. It may be helpful to insert a Foley catheter into the urethra to provide better identification. As would be expected, radical vulvectomy is associated with more bleeding than simple vulvectomy. As the lower base of the vulva is approached on each side, the internal pudendal vessels come into view and should be ligated separately (Fig. 93). At the posterior introitus, to avoid trauma to the anorectal area the same care must be exercised as described for simple vulvectomy. Tevdek sutures are used. A No. 12 Cystocath catheter is used for suprapubic bladder drainage. The No. 12 Cystocath or Hemovac tubes are employed for suction drainage through separate puncture sites below the base of the vulva on each side. A tight dressing is applied. In contrast to simple vulvectomy, prophylactic antibiotics are begun at the time of operation.

Postoperative Considerations. Postoperative care is between that applied for simple vulvectomy and that applied for radical vulvectomy with lymphadenectomy. Prophylactic antibiotics are continued for five days. Anticoagulants are not given. Suction tubes are removed when drainage becomes minimal. Except for the dressing around the suction tubes, the bulk of the dressing is left intact until it is necessary to remove it for bowel function; ambulation is encouraged after removal of the dressing. Voiding is not permitted until the 10th postoperative day, and the suprapubic catheter is removed on the following day. The 2–0 Tevdek sutures may be removed on the 14th postoperative day before discharge from the hospital, but the No. 1 Tevdek sutures and any sutures placed under tension are removed in the office four weeks after operation.

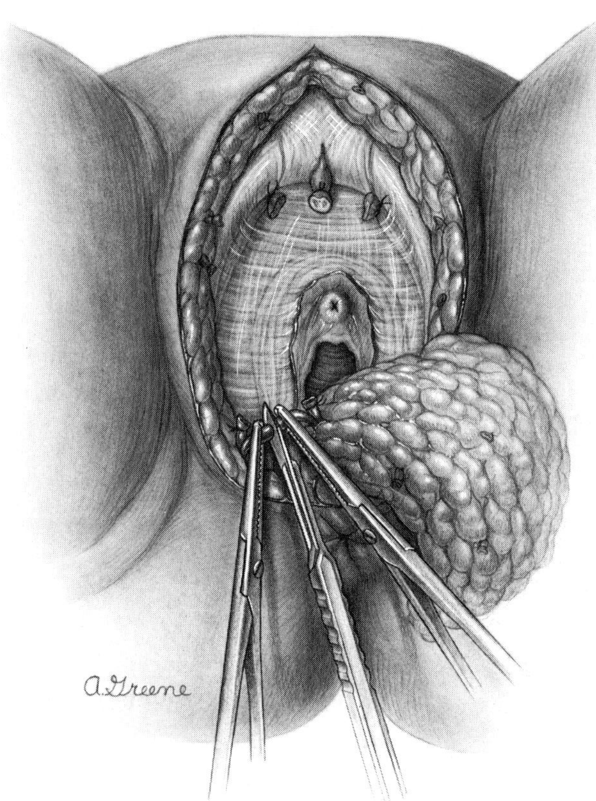

Figure 93.   Radical vulvectomy without lymphadenectomy. The skin and adjacent fat are excised widely down to the fascia, and the internal pudendal vessels are ligated.

Radical Vulvectomy and Lymphadenectomy

Comments. The optimum adequate surgical treatment for invasive carcinoma of the vulva has been radical vulvectomy with inguinal and deep pelvic lymphadenectomy. Green's classic reports of 1958 advocated this approach in achieving the maximum chance of cure. Way of England (1960) had been more radical only in advocating wider skin excision; this advice is wise when nodes are involved just beneath the skin. More recently Green (1978) reassessed his "adequate treatment" in the light of earlier diagnosis when the lesions are smaller and nodal metastases reduced. Morris (1977) presented data to support selective lymphadenectomy.

More conservative concepts of treatment than those mentioned have been recommended and should be considered, especially when dealing with the elderly poor-risk patient. For example, at the Radiumhemmet, Edsmyr (1962) combined local electrocoagulation and inguinal radiotherapy to achieve an absolute five-year patient survival rate of 72 per cent without and 30 per cent with metastases. Frischbier et al. (1971) obtained a five-year patient survival rate of 70 per cent for stages I and II tumors and 39 per cent for stages III and IV tumors using a dosage of 4,500 to 5,400 rads via 9 to 16 meV; they encountered serious complications in 8 per cent of their patients.

Figge and Gaudenz (1974), Parker et al. (1975), and Wharton et al. (1974) suggested radical vulvectomy without lymphadenectomy when dealing with well-differentiated squamous cell carcinoma less than 2 cm in greatest diameter with a depth of invasion less than 5 mm and without invasion of vascular channels. More recent reports by Kunschner et al. (1978) and Magrina et al. (1979) have stressed the need to individualize treatment of early cancer of the vulva. Magrina and associates observed only a 3 per cent incidence of positive nodes among patients with stage I lesions invading the stroma for 3 mm or less. However, Yazigi and coauthors (1978) challenged the wisdom of eliminating lymphadenectomy in stage I vulvar cancer, noting that in 10 of 103 women treated by vulvectomy alone inguinal node metastases later developed.

Foye and colleagues (1969) advocated local excision of the verrucous forms of vulvar carcinoma, and Schueller (1965) advocated the same approach for the pure form of basal cell carcinoma. To the contrary, in the good-risk patient, the surgeon should not hesitate to extend the scope of operation when necessary, for Krupp and associates (1975) reported a 30 per cent five-year survival rate when radical vulvectomy was combined with an exenterative procedure.

In summary, the surgeon should be wary of applying any standard therapy for vulvar carcinoma. Before treatment is considered, questions should be raised about the age and condition of the patient; the size, location, and depth of invasion of the lesion; the microscopic type and degree of differentiation; involvement of any vascular channels; and the presence of multiple lesions, palpable inguinal nodes, or contiguous urethral, anal, or vaginal involvement. These questions will be of greater practical importance, for increased accessibility of medical care should lead to earlier diagnosis in the future. The healthy woman with a reasonable life expectancy and stage I vulvar squamous carcinoma (2 cm lesion or less) should have the addition of femoral and inguinal lymphadenectomy if the tumor is poorly differentiated, if invasion is more than 3 mm deep, if vascular channels are involved with a negative metastatic series, or if suspicious lymph nodes are palpable. In regard to deep pelvic lymphadenectomy, the pathologist is asked to examine representative groin nodes while the vulvectomy site is being closed. If a node shows metastatic carcinoma, the groin incisions can be reprepared and opened in minutes to permit extension of the lymphadenectomy to the deep pelvis. As to the benefits of a conservative skin incision and of selective lymphadenectomy for unilateral lesions, I urge the reader to review in detail the reports of Green (1978) and Morris (1977), respectively.

A candidate for such radical surgery is admitted to a private room, which should be air conditioned in warm weather (cool dehumidified air is conducive to better healing of the wound). The customary radiograph of the chest, electrocardiogram, and hematologic and metastatic surveys are carried out with medical consultation as required. The patient is cross-matched for 5 units of blood. Subcutaneous heparin in a dose of 5,000 units is administered every 12 hours beginning the day before operation and continuing through the fifth day after operation. While radical vulvectomy with lymphadenectomy is not a difficult operation, it is tedious and may require up to five or six hours to perform. Therefore, it is wise to start operating early in the day.

Technique. The patient is placed in the supine position with the legs abducted 10 degrees and slightly overextended. A Foley catheter is placed in the bladder, and the lower part of the abdomen and upper thighs are prepared with povidone-iodine solution and draped. A crescent-shaped incision is made from one anterosuperior iliac spine to the other. A lower incision forms a narrow wedge of skin to be excised with the specimen (Fig. 94).

The subcutaneous fat is excised for several centimeters above the line of incision and for a wide area inferior to the lower incision to include the field of the inguinal and upper femoral lymph nodes. If any evidence is seen of lymphadenopathy adherent to the skin, a wide excision of skin is carried out in this area. The fat is cleaned off the fascia. The inferomedial aspect of the inguinal dissection is clarified by identifying the saphenous vein, which is divided and doubly ligated with 3–0 silk (Fig. 94, *inset*).

The fascia over the medial aspect of the sartorius muscle is incised and placed under tension as the dissection is carried into the femoral canal. Beware of the nerves, which are lateral and slightly deeper than the femoral artery. The vascular sheaths are opened, and the fat and nodes are easily cleaned off the vessels. Small arteries are divided and ligated near their origin from the femoral artery, most notably the external pudendal artery. The great saphenous vein is then divided at its junction with the femoral vein and is doubly ligated. The fat and nodes are pushed medially and freed from the underlying fascia until the vulva is reached (Fig. 95). In the process, the round ligament is identified and ligated at the external inguinal ring; if a fascial defect is present, it is closed with simple silk sutures. If the skin flaps over the groin can be approximated with only slight tension, the sartorius muscle should not be transplanted to cover the femoral vessels, for such a procedure only adds to the trauma of the operation and creates more dead space. Long suction tubes are placed above the incision in the groin through separate sites. Large Silastic tubes, polyethylene tubes (Hemovac), or No. 8 French rubber catheters may be used; whichever is chosen, small multiple openings should be made in the suction tube or catheter at intervals for its full length beneath the skin. Simple Tevdek sutures are used to approximate the skin, the size of the suture varying from 2–0 to 1 according to the tension of the wound (Fig. 96). The same steps are now repeated on the opposite groin, and the large bundle of dissected tissue is rolled medially and wrapped in a wet towel.

The patient is positioned for the vulvectomy. The Foley catheter is removed, and the area is reprepared with povidone-iodine solution and redraped. The radical vulvectomy is performed as described in the previous section (Fig. 97). A No. 12 Cystocath catheter is placed into the bladder for suprapubic drainage at the end of the vulvectomy. After the specimen is removed and while the vulvectomy site is being closed, the pathologist is asked to examine representative nodes. If metastatic carcinoma is found in the nodes, the patient is placed again in the supine position, and the incision is reopened. An incision is made through the external oblique aponeurosis parallel to the inguinal ligament, extending from the external inguinal ring to below the anterosuperior iliac spine. The internal oblique and transversalis muscles are divided in the same direction, and the inferior epigastric vessels are individually divided and ligated (Fig. 98).

The round ligament is divided after ligation, and the retroperitoneal space is easily exposed by manually deflecting the somewhat bulging peritoneal cavity with the adjacent ureter toward the midline. The fatty tissue and nodes adjacent to the external iliac vessel are gently and carefully removed up to the common iliac vessels. The forefinger and middle finger are used to begin to free the bundle of fatty tissue and nodes from the obturator space, in the process skeletonizing the obturator nerve. The remaining attachments of this bundle are severed with the dissecting scissors (Fig. 99). The internal oblique-transversalis muscles are approximated with horizontal mattress 1–0 chromic catgut or polyglycolic acid sutures, and the external oblique aponeurosis is closed with simple 3–0 silk sutures. The femoral canal is reduced by suturing the adjacent ligament to the underlying fascia as necessary to prevent the occurrence of a femoral hernia. Suction catheters are readjusted, and the incisions are closed again with Tevdek sutures (Fig. 100).

Postoperative Considerations. Drainage tubes are connected to low continuous suction, which is continued until drainage is minimal. Antibiotics are given for seven days in the form of intravenous sodium cephalothin, 1 gm every six hours, or intramuscularly administered tetracycline, 100 mg every eight hours for two days, followed by the oral form of the drug in a dose of 500 mg every six hours.

Intravenous fluids are continued for five days. Subcutaneous heparin (5,000 units) is administered every 12 hours for five days. The purpose of continuing intravenous fluids is to delay bowel elimination and contamination of the operative site. If blood loss through the drainage tubes is excessive, giving heparin is deferred for 48 hours. The foot of the bed is elevated 10 degrees. After several days, the patient is allowed to ambulate but not to sit up in a chair. These measures, together with the heparin, are aimed at reducing venous thrombosis — the main threat to life in the postoperative period. Suprapubic bladder drainage (No. 12 Cystocath) is continued for two weeks. Although the fine sutures may be removed at two weeks, the large tension sutures are not removed until approximately four weeks after operation, which may be after discharge from the hospital.

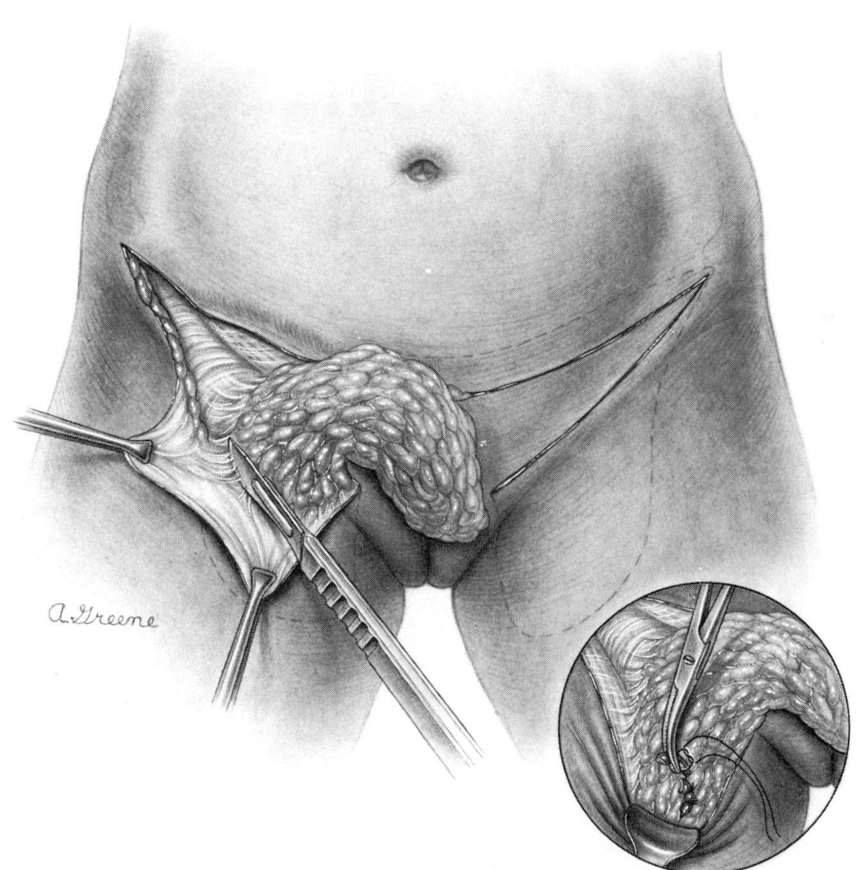

Figure 94. Radical vulvectomy and lymphadenectomy. A crescent-shaped incision is made from one antero-superior spine to the other, outlining a narrow wedge of skin to be excised. *Inset,* The saphenous vein is divided and doubly ligated at the inferomedial aspect of the inguinal dissection.

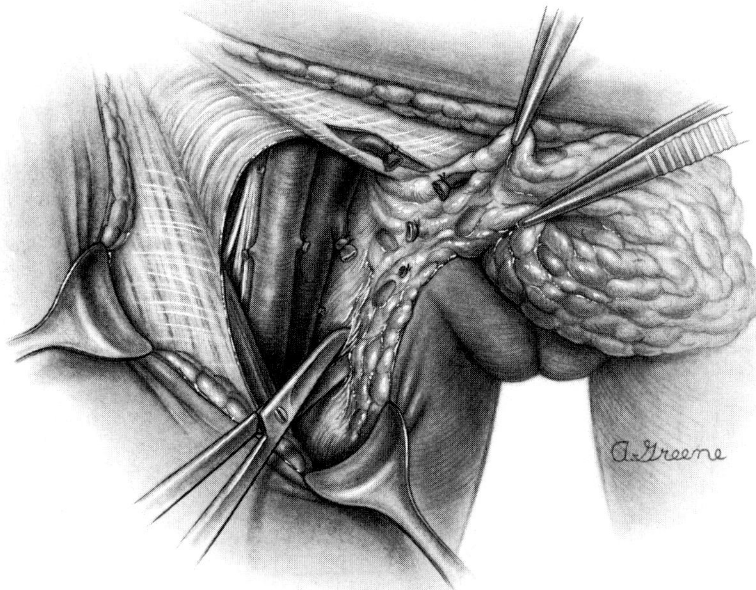

Figure 95. Radical vulvectomy and lymphadenectomy. The fat and nodes are freed from the underlying fascia and pushed medially toward the vulva. The round ligament is ligated at the external inguinal ring.

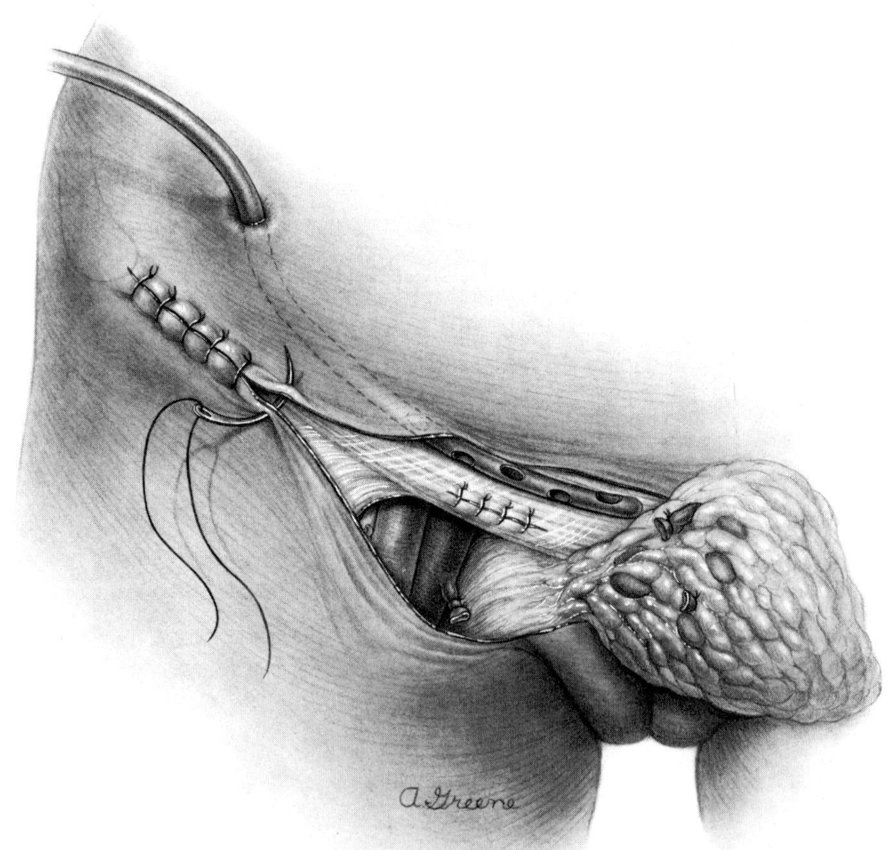

Figure 96. Radical vulvectomy and lymphadenectomy. Suction catheters are placed, and the skin is approximated with simple Tevdek sutures.

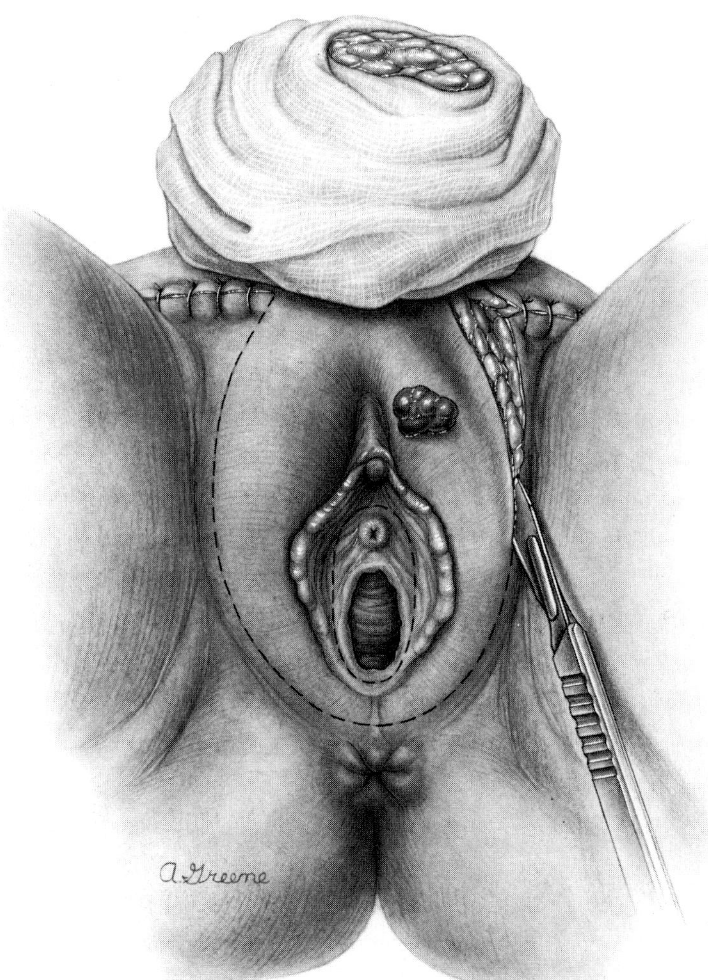

Figure 97. Radical vulvectomy and lymphadenectomy. The patient is positioned for radical vulvectomy.

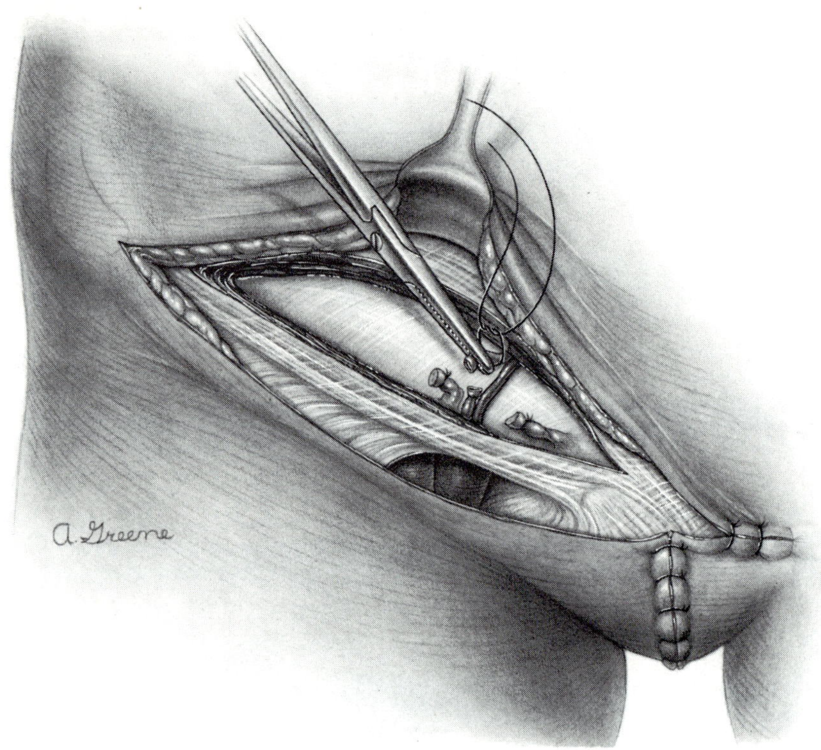

Figure 98. Radical vulvectomy and lymphadenectomy. If metastatic cancer is found in the groin nodes, the patient is returned to the supine position, sutures are removed, and an incision is made through the external oblique aponeurosis parallel to the inguinal ligament. The internal oblique and transversalis muscles are divided, and the epigastric vessels are divided and ligated.

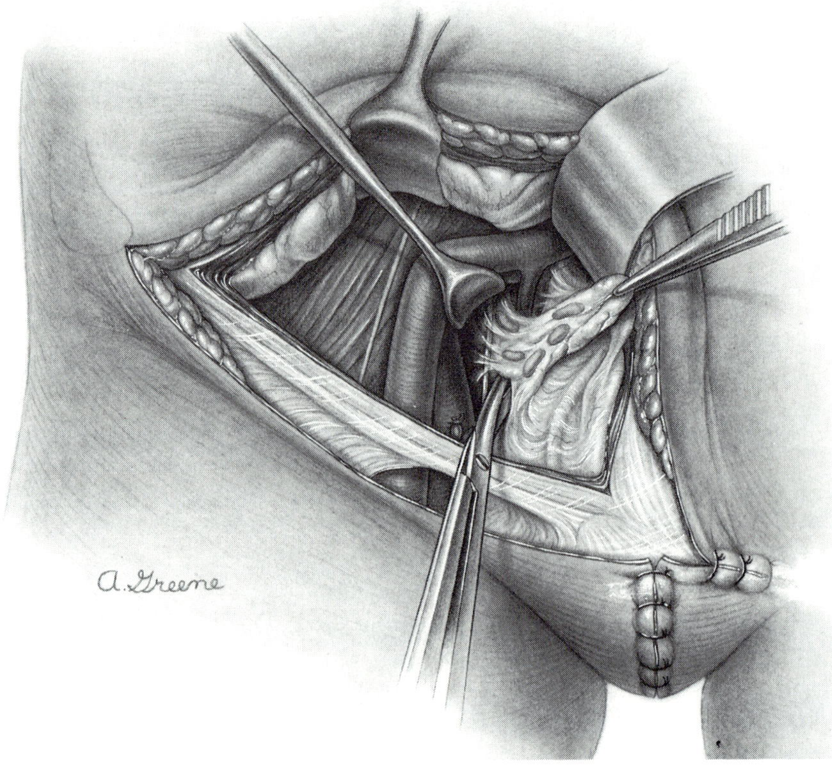

Figure 99. Radical vulvectomy and lymphadenectomy. The bladder, peritoneum, and attached ureter are pushed upward and medially to permit easy removal of tissue and nodes adjacent to the external iliac and common iliac vessels. The tissue and nodes in the obturator fossa are first freed by finger dissection and then carefully removed by sharp dissection, taking care not to injure the obturator nerve or the vessels on the floor of the fossa.

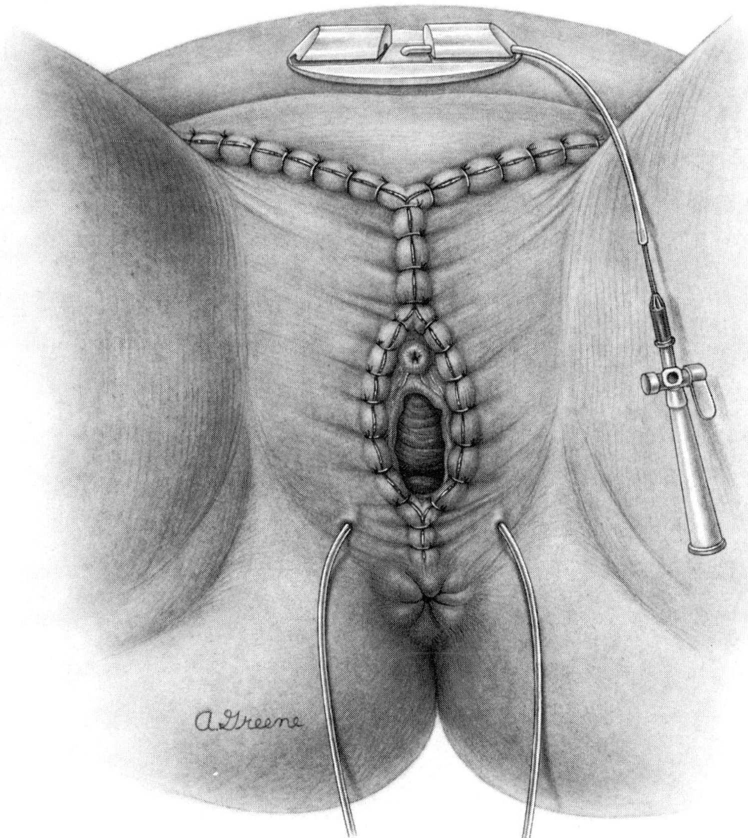

Figure 100.   Radical vulvectomy and lymphadenectomy. The incision is closed in layers, and the skin is reapproximated, leaving the suction catheters (bilateral groin and bilateral base of vulva) and suprapubic catheter in place.

Selected Bibliography

COMPLICATIONS AND MANAGEMENT

Amirikia, H, Evans, TN: Ten-year review of hysterectomies: trends, indications, and risks. Am J Obstet Gynecol 134:431–437 (June 15), 1979.

Copenhaver, EH: Vaginal hysterectomy: an analysis of indications and complications among 1,000 operations. Am J Obstet Gynecol 84:123–128 (July 1), 1962.

Ellsworth, HS, Harris, JW, McQuarrie, HG, et al.: Prolapse of the fallopian tube following vaginal hysterectomy. JAMA 224:891–892 (May 7), 1973.

Gray, LA: Views and reviews: indications, technics, and complications of vaginal hysterectomy. Obstet Gynecol 28:714–722 (Nov), 1966.

Kass, EH: Bacteriuria and the diagnosis of infections of the urinary tract: with observations on the use of methionine as a urinary antiseptic. Arch Intern Med 100:709–714 (Nov), 1957.

Ledger, WJ, Child, MA: The hospital care of patients undergoing hysterectomy: an analysis of 12,026 patients from Professional Activity Study. Am J Obstet Gynecol 117:423–433 (Oct 1), 1973.

Mattingly, RF: Te Linde's Operative Gynecology. 5th ed, Philadelphia, J B Lippincott Co, 1977, 871 pp.

Osborne, NG, Wright, RC, Dubay, M: Preoperative hot conization of the cervix: a possible method to reduce postoperative febrile morbidity following vaginal hysterectomy. Am J Obstet Gynecol 133:374–378 (Feb 15), 1979.

Pratt, JH, Scherman, Q: Morbidity in vaginal hysterectomy. Am J Obstet Gynecol 67:1323–1337 (June), 1954.

Schwarz, RH: Aerobes and anaerobes in postoperative infections. The Female Patient 75–78 (March), 1978.

Swartz, WH: Prophylaxis of minor febrile and major infectious morbidity following hysterectomy. Obstet Gynecol 54:284–288 (Sept), 1979.

Symmonds, RE: Prevention and management of genitourinary fistula. JCE Ob/Gyn 21:13–24 (June), 1979.

Thomsen, RJ: Prophylactic antibiotics for vaginal surgery: a historical addendum. Am J Obstet Gynecol 125:270–271 (May 15), 1976.

Thompson, JD: Urinary fistulas. Presented at the Symposium on Gynecology in honor of Richard W. Te Linde, MD, Atlanta, Georgia, Oct 14–15, 1977.

Zinman, LM, Libertino, JA, Roth, RA: Management of operative ureteral injury. Urology 12:290–303 (Sept), 1978.

MINOR VULVOVAGINAL SURGERY

Anderson, DG, Eaton, CJ, Galinkin, LJ, et al.: The cytologic diagnosis of endometrial adenocarcinoma. Am J Obstet Gynecol 125:376–388 (June 1), 1976.

Copenhaver, EH: A critical assessment of culdoscopy. Surg Clin North Am 50:713–718 (June), 1970.

Speroff, L (moderator): Is there a best way to do midtrimester abortions? Contemp Ob/Gyn 13:106–141 (May), 1979.

Woodruff, JD, Babaknia, A: Local alcohol injection of the vulva: discussion of 35 cases. Obstet Gynecol 54:512–514 (Oct), 1979.

MAJOR VULVOVAGINAL SURGERY

Colpocleisis

Copenhaver, EH: Surgical management of complete prolapse of the uterus and vagina. Surgical Practice of the Lahey Clinic. Philadelphia, W B Saunders Co, 1962, pp 689–694.

Copenhaver, EH: Abnormalities of pelvic support. In Lewis-Walters Practice of Surgery. Vol 10, Chapter 21, Hagerstown, Maryland, W F Prior Co, Inc, 1966, pp 1–30.

Correction of Stress Incontinence

Copenhaver, EH: Pubococcygeoplasty in the treatment of stress incontinence of urine. Lahey Clin Found Bull 27:58–61 (April-June), 1978.

Copenhaver, EH, Iliya, FA: Treatment of urinary stress incontinence — a current appraisal. Surg Clin North Am 45:765–773 (June), 1965.

Green, TH, Jr.: Urinary stress incontinence: differential diagnosis, pathophysiology, and management. Am J Obstet Gynecol 122:368–400 (June 1), 1975.

Obrink, A: Pubococcygeal repair ad modum Ingelman-Sundberg: a retrospective investigation with 10–20 years time of observation. Acta Obstet Gynecol Scand 56:391–397, 1977.

Tauber, R: Prevention of recurrences in the surgical treatment of urinary incontinence. Obstet Gynecol 23:104–106 (Jan), 1964.

Vaginal Hysterectomy

Copenhaver, EH: Vaginal hysterectomy: technique and operative complications. Surgical Practice of the Lahey Clinic. Philadelphia, W B Saunders Co, 1962, pp 681–688.

Copenhaver, EH: Vaginal hysterectomy: an analysis of indications and complications among 1,000 operations. Am J Obstet Gynecol *84*:123–128 (July 1), 1962.

Copenhaver, EH: Observations concerning blood loss during vaginal hysterectomy. Obstet Gynecol *24*:385–388 (Sept), 1964.

Copenhaver, EH: Abnormalities of pelvic support. *In* Lewis-Walters Practice of Surgery. Vol 10, Chapter 21, Hagerstown, Maryland, W F Prior Co, Inc, 1966, pp 1–30.

Revision of Congenital Malformations

Evans, TN: The artificial vagina. Am J Obstet Gynecol *99*:944–951 (Dec 1), 1967.

Farber, M, Marchant, DJ: Reconstructive surgery for congenital atresia of the uterine cervix. Fertil Steril *27*:1277–1282 (Nov), 1976.

Jones, HW, Jr.: An anomaly of the external genitalia in female patients with exstrophy of the bladder. Am J Obstet Gynecol *117*:748–756 (Nov 15), 1973.

Jones, HW, Jr., Wilkins, L: Gynecological operations in 94 patients with intersexuality: implications concerning the endocrine theory of sexual differentiation. Am J Obstet Gynecol *82*:1142–1153 (Nov), 1961.

Maciulla, GJ, Heine, MW, Christian, CD: Functional endometrial tissue with vaginal agenesis. J Reprod Med *21*:373–376 (Dec), 1978.

Niver, DH, Barrette, G, Jewelewicz, R: Congenital atresia of the uterine cervix and vagina: three cases. Fertil Steril *33*:25–29 (Jan), 1980.

Weed, JC, McKee, DM: Vulvoplasty in cases of exstrophy of the bladder. Obstet Gynecol *43*:512–516 (April), 1974.

Williams, EA: Congenital absence of the vagina: a simple operation for its relief. J Obstet Gynecol Brit Comm *71*:511–512 (Aug), 1964.

Revision of Narrowed Introitus

Scott, JW, Gilpin, CR, Vence, CA: Vulvectomy, introital stenosis, and Z plasty. Am J Obstet Gynecol *85*:132–133 (Jan 1), 1963.

Vulvectomy

Edsmyr, F: Carcinoma of vulva: an analysis of 560 patients with histologically verified squamous cell carcinoma. Acta Radiol Suppl *217*:1–135, 1962.

Figge, DC, Gaudenz, R: Invasive carcinoma of the vulva. Am J Obstet Gynecol *119*:382–395 (June 1), 1974.

Foye, G, Marsh, MR, Minkowitz, S: Verrucous carcinoma of the vulva. Obstet Gynecol *34*:484–488 (Oct), 1969.

Frischbier, HJ, Thomsen, K: Treatment of cancer of the vulva with high energy electrons. Am J Obstet Gynecol *111*:431–435 (Oct 1), 1971.

Green, TH, Jr., Ulfelder, H, Meigs, JV: Epidermoid carcinoma of the vulva: an analysis of 238 cases. I. Etiology and diagnosis. II. Therapy and end results. Am J Obstet Gynecol *75*:834–847, 848–864 (April), 1958.

Green, TH, Jr.: Carcinoma of the vulva: a reassessment. Obstet Gynecol *52*:462–469 (Oct), 1978.

Krupp, PJ, Lee, FY, Bohm, JW, et al.: Therapy of advanced epidermoid carcinoma of vulva. Report of 13 patients, with review of recent literature. Obstet Gynecol *46*:433–438 (Oct), 1975.

Kunschner, A, Kanbour, AI, David, B: Early vulvar carcinoma. Am J Obstet Gynecol *132*:599–606 (Nov 15), 1978.

Magrina, JF, Webb, MJ, Gaffey, TA, et al.: Stage I squamous cell cancer of the vulva. Am J Obstet Gynecol *134*:453–459 (June 15), 1979.

Morris, JM: A formula for selective lymphadenectomy: its application to cancer of the vulva. Obstet Gynecol *50*:152–158 (Aug), 1977.

Parker, RT, Duncan, I, Rampone, J, et al.: Operative management of early invasive epidermoid carcinoma of the vulva. Am J Obstet Gynecol *123*:349–355 (Oct 15), 1975.

Schueller, EF: Basal cell cancer of the vulva. Am J Obstet Gynecol *93*:199–208 (Sept 15), 1965.

Way, S: Carcinoma of the vulva. Am J Obstet Gynecol *79*:692–697 (April), 1960.

Wharton, JT, Gallager, S, Rutledge, FN: Microinvasive carcinoma of the vulva. Am J Obstet Gynecol *118*:159–162 (Jan 15), 1974.

Yazigi, R, Piver, MS, Tsukada, Y: Microinvasive carcinoma of the vulva. Obstet Gynecol *51*:368–370 (March), 1978.

Index

Note: Page numbers in *italics* refer to illustrations.